# PAIN, DEATH AND TAXES

A Proven Pain Patient Survival Guide

William E. Ackerman III MD

PAIN, DEATH AND TAXES

A Proven Pain Patient Survival Guide

Copyright © 2017 by William E. Ackerman III MD

All rights reserved. No part of this book may be reproduced or transmitted in any form or by any means without written permission of the author.

This book is dedicated to my significant other, my family, and my staff and to my patients whose frequent questions inspired the content for this book.

# Acknowledgments

I wish to acknowledge my patients. Their questions that they asked concerning their pain prompted the writing of this book. If a patient has a basic understanding of their pain pathology, it helps he or she cope better with the pain and helps the treating physician better understand their suffering and ultimately provide better care.

# Foreword

Pain management has become an important and growing medical specialty. There is an attitude among individuals suffering from chronic pain that they are no longer willing to suffer pain in silence. Dramatic changes have been made with respect to the understanding of the anatomy and physiology of many painful entities over the past two decades. New drugs and other modalities are being introduced with increasing frequently. A pain patient needs to partner with his or her doctor in order to obtain pain relief. This book gives a pain patient the basic proven information necessary to rationally discuss his or her pain with the treating physician. Many primary care physicians have no or minimal pain training. This book will furthermore, enable a patient to derive basic pain management knowledge that may be helpful when he or she communicates with their pain management physician.

## Table of Contents

1. PAIN OVERVIEW .................................................................. 1
2. PAIN PERCEPTION (A computer model) .......................... 9
3. PAIN INPUT ......................................................................... 15
4. PAIN RELIEF ....................................................................... 21
5. PAIN DIAGNOSIS ................................................................ 25
6. PAIN DOCTORS .................................................................. 31
7. OPIOID MEDICATIONS ..................................................... 35
8. ADDICTION ........................................................................ 41
9. NON-STEROIDAL MEDICATIONS ................................... 45
10. MUSCLE RELAXANTS ..................................................... 51
11. NEUROPATHIC PAIN ....................................................... 57
12. ANTIDEPRESSANT DRUGS ............................................ 63
13. TOPICAL PAIN RELIEVERS ........................................... 69
14. PHYSICAL THERAPY ...................................................... 79
15. CHIROPRACTIC MEDICINE ........................................... 85
16. PSYCHOLOGY AND PAIN .............................................. 89
17. LOW BACK PAIN .............................................................. 93
18. NECK PAIN ........................................................................ 99
19. FIBROMYALGIA .............................................................. 103
20. MYOFASCIAL PAIN ........................................................ 109
21. HEADACHES ................................................................... 115
22. NEUROPATHY ................................................................ 123
23. ARTHRITIS ...................................................................... 129
24. OSTEOPOROSIS .............................................................. 137

25. SHINGLES ..................................................................................141
26. RSD ........................................................................................147
27. VASCULAR DISEASE ............................................................153
28. CANCER PAIN .......................................................................159
29. CHEST PAIN ...........................................................................165
30. ABDOMINAL PAIN ...............................................................173
31. ELDERLY PAIN .....................................................................181
32. GENDER PAIN .......................................................................187

# 1. PAIN OVERVIEW

The word computer refers to an object that can accept some input and produce some output. In fact, the human brain itself is a sophisticated computer. Your brain like a computer takes pain responses from your body and interprets these electrical activities as pain. In order to understand pain physiology you can compare electrical neurological activities with computer activities. Many pain patients request narcotic medications which affect the entire brain instead of focusing on decreasing pain impulses to the brain. The CPU, often just called the processor, is the computer component that contains the microprocessor. That microprocessor like the patient's brain is the heart of all the PC's operations and the performance of both hardware and software rely on the processor's performance. Your brain is like a computer in that it transfers electrical signals (pain and other impulses) to the brain. Narcotics can anesthetize the brain which in turn can decrease pain intensities but can also cause drunkenness, sedation etc. These effects can decrease a patient's ability to function in a normal manner.

Data transmission is the process of sending digital or analog data over a communication medium to one or more computing, network, communication or electronic devices. It enables the transfer and communication of devices in a point-to-point, point-to-multipoint and multipoint-to-multipoint environment. The operating system is what allows your computer software to communicate with the computer hardware (nerves throughout your body). Analog or analogue transmission is a transmission method of conveying voice, data, image, signal or video information using a continuous signal which varies in amplitude, phase, or some other property in proportion to that of a variable. Your body also transfers pain impulses in a similar fashion. In telecommunications, parallel transmission is the simultaneous transmission of the signal elements of a character or other entity of data. In digital communications, parallel transmission is the simultaneous transmission of related signal elements over two or more separate paths. Multiple electrical wires are used which can transmit multiple bits simultaneously, which allows for higher data transfer rates than can be achieved with serial transmission. Your body, through similar physiologic mechanisms does the same tasks.

Patients need to understand that pain can be decreased by decreasing pain signal intensity input to your central pain processor which is your brain. You do not have to decrease total brain activity. A computer is an electronic machine that processes information like a computer processor. Taking in information is called input, storing information is known as memory, handling this information is known as processing, and emitting results of the input information is called output. Even the fastest processor needs a buffer to store information while it's being processed. The RAM is to the CPU as a countertop is to a cook: It serves as the place where the information and brain processing tools you're working such as the midbrain with wait until you need to do an activity such as walking, bending etc. to avoid increasing your pain. Both a fast CPU and an ample amount of RAM are necessary for a speedy PC processing.

The brain is a processer that has a cortex which functions as a computer drive. A drive is a device intended to store data when it's not in use. Your brain stores data in your brain related to previous life experiences. Your brain receives input from the midbrain as well. Your computer receives input from your body. Your nerves and senses deliver input to your brain like a keyboard and mouse so that your brain can process this information. Your computer probably stores all your documents and files on a hard-drive which is a large magnetic memory. But smaller, computer-based devices like digital cameras and cellphones use other kinds of storage such as flash memory cards. Your computer has an LCD screen capable of revealing high-resolution graphics, and probably also stereo loudspeakers. Your brain has a mind which can perform the same tasks.

The concept that pain results from mechanically and chemically caused physical changes that become more and more difficult to reverse is well-accepted throughout Medicine. Pain should be described as an abstract model of pain based on electrical values: sensors (free nerve endings), wires (axons/nerves) and the perceptron (spinal cord and brain). Pain is described as either nociceptive (normal working of pain fibers), neuropathic (misfiring of axons/nerves), or central dysfunctions (central nervous system), the latter includes the pain pathways in the spinal cord and the brain. Neuropathic pain is related to nerve (wire) dysfunction and treatment must, concentrate on reversing that pathology. Be aware that more than one of the basic mechanisms becomes active (i.e. nociceptive pain may progress to neuropathic pain and then to central pain), the physician can address one mechanism at a time by choosing treatment methods that are logically most effective and logistically most convenient. Without visible tissue changes, there may not be a peripheral pain generator, leaving neuropathic and/or central pain as the probable cause. Ultimately, there must always be a mechanism whereby some pathology or dysfunction causes the perception of pain. Chronic pain most likely encompasses all three types of pain: nociceptive, neuropathic, and central.

The ancient Greeks such as Aristotle were the first individuals who believed that pain was derived from various nerves in the body. The exact cause of pain was unknown to them. Unfortunately, not unlike ancient times, the diagnosis and treatment of many chronic painful conditions today remains mostly guesswork. Pain medicine is for the most part subjectively based, because pain is a subjective symptom while other medical specialties are based upon objective medical evidence. Pain in general is not bad. Pain is a protective mechanism that warns you that your body has something wrong at some location. The sensation of pain tells you to stop activity or to at least slow down your activity. For example if you sprain your ankle, your pain is a warning for you not to put weight on that leg. The International Association for the Study of Pain defines pain as" an unpleasant sensory and emotional experience associated with tissue injury as a result of trauma (e.g. bone fracture) or disease (e.g. cancer, shingles).

Pain has psychological effects in some instances especially when pain is severe. Pain may cause anxiety and depression. Acute pain is associated with injury, bone fractures, surgery or sprains and strains. Once these entities have healed sometimes, the pain continues. Arthritis is another example of chronic pain. Arthritic pain is caused by continuous joint destruction. However, once the pain becomes chronic, your pain it becomes a problem. Not only does pain become a personal problem but pain can become a social problem with creation of family problems, loss of self-esteem and lost wages. Fibromyalgia patients have alterations in CNS anatomy, physiology, and chemistry that potentially contribute to the symptoms experienced by these patients.Pain impulses are in essence, electrical signals that travel from various areas of your body such as the extremities, heart, appendix etc.

to the spinal cord and eventually reach the brain where the pain signals are processed like data in a computer. The brain is like a computer hard drive, which stores painful experiences that ultimately results in the suffering associated with chronic pain. Pain is produced by unpleasant stimuli to nerve endings throughout the body which include chemical, extreme heat cold and mechanical injury. These nerve endings are silent until mechanical, heat or cold injures tissue. In order to experience pain we need these pain receptors and the nerve fibers that transmit pain to the spinal cord and then to the brain.

Nerves, which conduct pain impulses to the spinal cord, are composed of neurons (nerve cells) that make up nerve fibers that form neurons. Two common pain fibers are the C fibers and the A-delta fibers. A-delta fibers conduct fast onset sharp pain impulses. The C fibers conduct slow onset dull, aching or burning pain. If you hit your finger with a hammer, you will experience a sudden pain response followed by a dull pain response. A neuron is an electrically excitable cell in the nervous system that processes and transmits information. Neurons are the significant core components of your brain and spinal cord as well as your peripheral nerves. Neurons are the building blocks of nerves. In other words, multitudes of neurons are necessary to form a nerve. Nerves that exist outside of your central nervous system are called ganglia. Various ganglia may form a plexus. An example of a plexus is your celiac plexus. Sometimes this plexus is blocked with numbing medicine or phenol or alcohol to relieve severe abdominal pain. Surgery may also be necessary on occasion for pain relief.

Action potentials generated by the neuron initiate pain signals. An action potential begins after a depolarization (a change in the electrical activity within the neuron) such that it could cause a membrane transitory modification, turning prevalently permeable to sodium ions more than to potassium ions. Sodium permeability can cause an action potential. Following an acute injury, AMPA receptors are stimulated which cause sharp pain. Receptors (areas in the body where biochemicals or drugs attach) are present in the spinal cord are called NMDA (N-methyl-D-aspartate) receptors and cause chronic pain. When these NMDA receptors are chemically and/or electrically stimulated, pain becomes more severe and this severe pain is maintained which implies that the pain does not decrease. The brain is responsible for the suffering associated with pain. Pain results in bodily responses especially with respect to the cardio-vascular system (heart rate increases, blood pressure increases, renal arteries constrict etc.). When pain is severe, the brain can cause the body to increase both the heart rate and blood pressure. Severe pain can also result in profuse sweating as well as nausea and vomiting. Pain signals from areas in the body reach the brain by four processes (transduction, transmission, modulation and perception).

Pain signals enter the back of your spinal cord. They cross over to the other side. The pain impulses will then proceed upwards to go to your brain. It is important to know that pain signals can be dampened by structures and chemicals that exist in your spinal cord. Pain signals are transmitted from the site of injury as action potentials. Electrical and/or chemical activity between the neuron dendrites and axons propagate the axon potentials. Axons carry pain fibers away from your neuron and direct them to the dendrites of the next neuron through synapses until they terminate in your brain or spinal cord. They form synapses or clefts between the axon and dendrite. The synapse has chemicals in the axon nerve ending. These chemicals allow communication between the neurons. Drugs are chemicals that can interrupt the communication between the neurons.

You need to understand that pain signals cross to the opposite side from the injury and therefore travel to the opposite side of your brain. It is important to understand these processes in order to understand how your pain can be treated effectively. Transduction is a process where electrical signals originate in the nerve endings throughout your body. These impulses are chemically, mechanically and/or thermally mediated and transmitted to your spinal cord where they can be modulated and then sent to your brain. Tissue injury or disease (including arthritis) cause the body to release biochemicals called prostaglandins. Prostaglandins themselves do not cause pain. Prostaglandins do however sensitize pain receptors to other chemicals in the body, which facilitate the transmission of pain impulses. Nonsteroidal drugs like ibuprofen decrease the number of prostaglandins produced in your body and may in a decrease in your pain perception. Topical creams such as Ben Gay can decrease the process of transduction at the nerve endings.

Transmission is a process where pain signals are transported to the spinal cord. Nerves in body tissues transmit electrical impulses to the spinal cord. Nerve blocks with anesthetics like Novicaine can interrupt the transmission of pain impulses to the spinal cord. Once pain impulses reach the spinal cord they are modulated or changed by chemicals and nerves that inhibit or lessen the number of pain impulses from going up the spinal cord to your brain. Fibers called internuncial fibers are present within the spinal cord that can decrease pain transmission by filtering pain nerve impulses. The brain can send impulses back to these pain control fibers within the spinal cord to decrease the number of impulses that reach the pain perception center of the brain. This is the basis of hypnosis. The spinal cord acts like a transformer to intensify or decrease the intensity of pain impulses. Narcotics and anticonvulsants can modulate pain impulses within the spinal cord. Finally, pain impulses reach the brain where you perceive pain and this information is stored in your brain similar to a computer. Narcotics can "numb" your brain to decrease the effects of the pain impulses on your brain by decreasing the intensity of these impulses. Higher brain centers determine how we respond to a painful stimulus. Melzak and Wall described this Gate Control Theory in 1965. Different types of nerve fibers (both pain and non-pain fibers) enter the spinal cord at the same time. Non-pain fibers essentially dilute out the number of pain impulses that

In order for you to hurt, pain-producing chemicals in your body tissue must stimulate pain fibers (Alpha-delta and C fibers). In general, the greater the tissue trauma, the more pain transmitting chemicals are produced and the worse the pain. When a stimulus such as heat produces, tissue injury chemicals are released at the site of nerve injury, which cause pain fibers to become hyperactive. These chemicals include bradykinin, histamine, substance p, acetylcholine, serotonin and histamine. These chemicals act at the nerve endings and ultimately send pain impulses to the spinal cord and brain. The nerves that conduct pain go to the spinal cord that allows pain signals to ultimately reach the brain. Areas of your body that have many pain receptors include the skin, the outer aspect of bone called the periosteum, ligaments, joints, teeth and gums and the cornea of the eye. Muscle also contains pain fibers but not as many per square meter (a measure of area) as the previously mentioned structures.

Where the pain nerves from your body enter your spinal cord, aspartic and glutamic acid are produced. These acids increase pain impulse generation. NMDA may be produced. GABA (gamma-aminobutyric acid) in the spinal cord on the other hand, decreases the number of pain impulses that reach the brain. GABA inhibits pain impulse transmission Norepinepherine and serotonin are two more chemicals in the spinal cord which attenuate the number of pain impulses which reach your brain. The brain and spinal cord regulate pain by the production of naturally occurring narcotic-like substances that decrease pain transmission in specific areas of the brain. These narcotic-like drugs are called enkephalins, dynorphins and beta-endorphins. Some of these substances also decrease pain transmission in the spinal cord. Enkephalins are located in areas of the brain related to pain modulation.

Remember that prostaglandins sensitize pain nerve endings to pain producing tissue chemicals. Antidepressant drugs like Elavil or Prozac decrease pain by increasing norepinephrine and serotonin in the spinal cord. As previously mentioned, these two substances decrease the number of pain impulses that reach the pain perception areas of the brain. Anticonvulsant drugs like gabapentin affect GABA and by enhancing GABA blood levels which in turn decreases the number of pain signals in your spinal cord that can go to your brain. Narcotic drugs also decrease pain impulse conduction in both the spinal cord and brain. Injections of numbing medicine (local anesthetics with steroids) can decrease pain in muscle and nerves in the arms, legs and the trunk of the body. There is an area of your brain that represents an area where you process pain signals like a computer. This area detects tissue injury and is a protective mechanism to alert you that something is wrong. A burn of the palm of your hand alerts your brain that tissue injury is occurring and initiates a reflex in your spinal cord to have you immediately remove your hand from the hot object. Without pain interpretation in your brain, you could sustain multiple bodily traumas and have no knowledge of its occurrence.

# 2. PAIN PERCEPTION (A computer model)

The previous chapter relates that the brain is like a computer because like a computer, our body/brain communicates and carries out functions through the use of electrical currents. Information travels from every part of our body to the brain and from the brain to the body. The brain is made up of many specialized areas that work together: The cortex is the outermost layer of brain cells. Thinking and voluntary movements begin in the cortex. The brain stem is between the spinal cord and the rest of the brain. Basic functions like breathing and sleep are controlled here. The basal ganglion is a cluster of structures in the center of the brain. The basal ganglia coordinate messages between multiple other brain areas. The cerebellum is at the base and the back of the brain. The cerebellum is responsible for coordination and balance. The cortex is the outer layer of the brain and is where you perceive your pain.

A computer is defined as an electronic device that processes data according to a set of instructions or commands, known as a program. The main memory is the memory that temporarily stores information while it is being sent to the CPU. It also helps break down the information to something the CPU can easily understand. Main memory can be thought of as "the bouncer" of the core, everything that happens goes through the main memory first. The main memory is often referred to as RAM, or random-access memory. In other words, the memory can be retrieved or written to anywhere in the memory. The computer does not have to go through all the information in the memory to get to the information at the very end. Think about old cassette tapes. To get to the next song, the current song needs to be either played all the way through or fast forwarded through; this kind of memory is called sequential memory. RAM is more like a CD.

The software of the computer is just a series of ones and zeros at the lowest level and cannot physically be touched and is usually stored on the hard drive of the computer. The software can be broken down into two general categories: the operating system and the applications. The operating system (OS) is the visual representation of the computer. The OS includes the desktop, start menu, icons, file view, etc. Hardware includes the physical parts of the computer and includes devices such as the monitor, keyboard, speakers, wires, chips, cables, plugs, disks, printers, mice, and many other items that can physically be touched. Hardware includes the physical parts of the computer and includes devices such as the monitor, keyboard, speakers, wires, chips, cables, plugs, disks, printers, mice, and many other items that can physically be touched. There are two categories of hardware that each contains two parts: the core (the central processing unit (CPU) and the main memory) and the peripherals (the input and output (I/O) devices and the secondary memory).

The core of a computer consists of the CPU and the main memory. The secondary memory is all other memory outside of the main memory that the computer accesses. Secondary memory is used for long-term storage and gets physically changed when files are saved or deleted. Common secondary memory devices are the hard drive, floppy disks, CD-ROMs, USB storage devices, and flash drives. These things hold the software (OS and Apps) that the main memory will access. The input and output (I/O) devices are how the user interacts with the computer. Without these devices, the computer would not be very helpful. The most common input devices are the keyboard and the mouse. In telecommunications, parallel transmission is the simultaneous transmission of the signal elements of a character or other entity of data. In digital communications, parallel transmission is the simultaneous transmission of related signal elements over two or more separate paths. Multiple electrical wires are used which can transmit multiple bits simultaneously, which allows for higher data transfer rates than can be achieved with serial transmission.

Another difference between main and secondary memory is that main memory is usually volatile and secondary is usually nonvolatile. This difference refers to the stored information and the power supply. Volatile means that information is deleted when the power is turned off whereas in the case of nonvolatile the information remains. One reason to believe it does is that, much like a computer, the brain functions as an input-output system. Stimuli received as input from sensory systems are processed and a corresponding response is generated. The human brain is incredibly complex. We still don't have a full understanding of how the brain works. Without this understanding, it's challenging to create a meaningful simulation of the brain. The computational theory of mind, in essence, says that your brain works like a computer. That is, it takes input from the outside world, and then performs algorithms to produce output in the form of mental state or action. In other words, it claims that the brain is an information processor where your mind is "software" that runs on the "hardware" of the brain.

The nervous system is an input-output system. For example, the nervous system takes sensory information such as visual data as input and also generates movement of the muscles as output. Second, the nervous system is functionally organized in a specific way such that it has specific capacities, such as generating conscious experience. Third, the brain is a feedback-control system: the nervous system controls an organism's behavior in response to its environment. Finally, the nervous system processes information: feedback-control can be performed because the brain's internal states correlate with external states. A synapse is basically brain neurons (nerve cells) communicating with one another via electrical or chemical signals. Human-Memory.net has some staggering figures relating to this topic. The source notes the average human brain contains about 100 billion neurons that can be connected to up to 10,000 other neurons. The most powerful computer known is the brain. The human brain possesses about 100 billion neurons with roughly 1 quadrillion ( 1 million billion) connections known as synapses wiring these cells together.

Computers do many things very well. They can perform complex calculations, and the fastest computers can crunch trillions of numbers each second. Humans make calculations in a way similar to digital computers. The human prefrontal cortex and basal ganglia appear to have two states similar to the binary systems in a computer. Things like emotion, self-awareness, ambition and self-preservation all rest within our brains. Computers don't experience these concepts.

Pain has been a major concern of humankind since the ancient times, and it remains one of the most important subjects of all health care professionals. Despite the obvious overwhelming clinical importance, the major advances in its diagnosis and therapy have been made only recently. "How do the sensory apparatus of the body and system of signal transmission relate to pain of peripheral origin?" is the topic of discussion. To do this, it is important to understand what constitutes the total pain experience. It consists of: 1) signal transduction at the peripheral receptor site, 2) signal conduction along the peripheral nerve, 3) pain modulation at the level of the spinal cord, 4) pain perception at the supraspinal site, and 5) the associated sensations, emotional reactions, and effective state. The signal transmission related to pain may be modified by various analgesic agents. Specific analgesic agent has a specific site of action, which may be at peripheral receptors, at peripheral nerves, at the level of the spinal cord, at supraspinal levels by activating descending inhibitory systems, or at more cephalad levels by reducing the affective component of pain.

Stimuli which cause pain are picked up by nociceptors and converted into nerve impulses, which travel to the brain. Pain information in the form of nerve impulses is carried from your foot to the spinal cord and from here it is relayed to the brain. Pain can be modified or modulated in the spinal cord. This means that pain can be enhanced or lessened or blocked completely. This modulation takes place in the dorsal horn of the spinal cord. Pain is interpreted and perceived in the brain. Pain is modulated by two primary types of drugs that work on the brain: analgesics and anesthetics. The term analgesic refers to a drug that relieves pain without loss of consciousness. The term central anesthesia refers to a drug that depresses the CNS. It is characterized by the absence of all perceptions of sensory modalities, including loss of consciousness without loss of vital functions.

The first pain modulator mechanism called the "Gate Control" theory was proposed by Melzack and Wall in the mid-1960s. The concept of the gate control theory is that non-painful input closes the gates to painful input, which results in prevention of the pain sensation from traveling to the CNS (i.e., non-noxious input [stimulation] suppresses pain). The gate control theory of pain modulation is based on presynaptic inhibition of pain information produced by mechanical stimulation, and provides the basic rationale for the TENS. The total pain experience in essence consists of: 1) signal transduction at the peripheral receptor site, 2) signal conduction along the peripheral nerve, 3) pain modulation at the level of the spinal cord, 4) pain perception at the supraspinal site, and 5) the associated sensations, emotional reactions, and effective state. The signal transmission related to pain may be modified by various analgesic agents. Specific analgesic agent has a specific site of action which may be at peripheral receptors, at peripheral nerves, at the level of the spinal cord, at supraspinal levels by activating descending inhibitory systems, or at more cephalad levels by reducing the affective component of pain.

The theory suggests that collaterals of the large sensory fibers carrying cutaneous sensory input activate inhibitory interneurons, which inhibit (modulate) pain transmission information carried by the pain fibers. Non-noxious input suppresses pain, or sensory input "closes the gate" to noxious input. The gate theory predicts that at the spinal cord level, non-noxious stimulation will produce presynaptic inhibition on dorsal root nociceptor fibers that synapse on nociceptors spinal neurons , and this presynaptic inhibition will block incoming noxious information from reaching the CNS (i.e., will close the gate to incoming noxious information). Acute pain can last a moment and rarely does it become chronic pain. Chronic pain persists for long periods. It is resistant to most medical treatments and cause severe problems. Even though the experience of pain varies from one person to the next; it is possible to categorize the different types of pain. When nerve fibers get damaged, the result can be chronic pain. Psychogenic pathology such as depression, anxiety, and other emotional problems can cause pain or make existing pain worse. Musculoskeletal pain is pain that affects the muscles, ligaments and tendons, and bones. Learn about the causes, symptoms, and treatments. Use your muscles incorrectly, too much, too little and you've acquired muscle pain.

A stroke, multiple sclerosis, or spinal cord injuries can result in chronic pain and burning syndromes from damage to brain regions. The Complex Regional Pain Syndrome is a baffling, intensely painful disorder that can develop from a seemingly minor injury, yet is believed to result from high levels of nerve impulses being sent to the affected disorder. Learn more about this disorder. Diabetes-Related Nerve Pain (Neuropathy) may occur if you have diabetes, and nerve damage can be a serious complication. This nerve complication can cause severe burning pain, especially at night. (Postherpetic Neuralgia), Shingles is a painful condition that arises from varicella-zoster, the same virus that causes chickenpox. Trigeminal Neuralgia is considered one of the most painful conditions in medicine.

The treatment of pain is guided by the history of the pain, its intensity, duration, aggravating and relieving conditions, and structures involved in causing the pain. In other words, there are multiple causes of pain. In order for a structure to cause pain, it must have a nerve supply, be susceptible to injury, and stimulation of the structure should cause pain. The concept behind most interventional procedures for treating pain is that there is a specific structure in the body with nerves of sensation that is generating the pain. Pain management has a role in identifying the precise source of the problem and isolating the optimal treatment. In order for a pain management physician to adequately treat your pain he/she must know a detailed history of your pain in order to make a correct diagnosis and to prescribe the correct treatment.

# 3. PAIN INPUT

Animal models have enhanced our understanding of pain mechanisms and make forward-looking statements as to our proximity to the development of effective mechanism-based treatments. Animal pain models have failed in some aspects as animal models cannot always be extrapolated to humans. Our computer model presumes doctors know where the pain originates. Pain is an unpleasant sensory and emotional experience following tissue injury. Your pain management can be expensive as well as ineffective if you do not communicate truthfully with you doctor. Different specialties in medicine practice pain medicine. Chiropractors practice pain management as well. Anesthesiologists manage your pain with injections. Physiatrists manage pain with heat, cold, etc. and do needle studies on you to see if you have nerve damage. Orthopedic and neurosurgeons can perform surgery on you. A neuro-surgeon can place a spinal morphine pump that directs morphine into your spinal fluid. All of these specialists can prescribe drugs to you for pain management. The effectiveness of psychosocial interventions for back pain in primary care has been established.

Pain input in processed in your brain as a result of signals from one or more parts of your body that are submitted to your brain for processing. As previously stated your brain is your CPU. Tissue inflammation, nerve compression, tissue injury, hyperactive nerves etc. can cause you to experience pain. As a result, a pain patient may require surgery (i.e. to remove a disc herniation), a muscle relaxant for muscle pain, and an anti-inflammatory medication for arthritic pain, an anti-elliptic for neuropathic pain or a narcotic-like drug for cancer pain. Your sensory information (pain responses) sent to your brain (your CPU) will determine the type of treatment that you will receive.

For thousands of years, doctors have been helping to relieve their patients' pain with a variety of medications and treatments. Like other areas of medicine, a new subset of doctors has become specialists in treating pain. The question that you should ask yourself is if any of the modalities such as heat, cold, injections, drugs etc. will actually stop your pain. The answer is no if your pain is chronic. Chronic pain is a disease. Your doctor will strive to provide you with a quality of life. If your pain is acute such as post-surgical pain, or after a fall on your hip you should expect significant pain relief. Chronic pain is that pain that persists after your body has healed. Nothing unfortunately will completely eliminate your pain.

The goal of pain management is to decrease your pain so that you can maintain your normal activities of daily living. This means that your pain should not interfere with your work, family or recreation. As a result, if you have chronic pain your goal and your doctor's goal should be to decrease your pain to a tolerable level. Pain management is expensive. Because nothing will completely stop your chronic pain, you will need to follow up frequently with your health care provider. Different treatments will be tried until you begin to have a reduction in your pain. When you see a specialist or go to a hospital or surgery center, if you have insurance, you will have to pay a co-payment to have a procedure or an examination performed. Because many pain treatments will not benefit you, it is necessary for you to become an informed consumer. You can do this by trying to understand what is causing your pain and what alternative modalities (such as chiropractic, herbs etc.) are available to you.

If you complain of pain to your primary care physician, your doctor may refer you to someone who only treats pain. This individual may have no or minimal training or may have extensive training. You must be aware that pain management can be an environment where essentially a practitioner in some situations needs only minimal credentials such as a medical license to do potentially harmful procedures to unsuspecting individuals suffering from excruciating pain. This can be a world where most procedures can be done in out-patient surgery centers to avoid the peer review scrutiny of a hospital medical staff. You must therefore, inquire if your practitioner is trained and certified in pain medicine. Approximately forty-eight million Americans suffer from chronic pain.

Americans spend over one hundred billion dollars annually on pain care. One-third of all adult Americans suffer from some degree of chronic pain. Over the counter annual analgesic costs amount to three billion dollars. Your pain treatment can bankrupt you. You must be able to identify the ethical pain treatment physicians and clinics as well as the "get rich" schemers. The cost of medical care is rapidly escalating. Employers may not be able to afford health insurance for their employees. The cost of pain management is contributing to the increase in health care costs and amounts to hundreds of thousands of dollars. As a result, there is considerable profit to be made by unethical health care providers that include hospitals as well as physicians. Unfortunately, along with many reputable excellent pain clinics many pain management centers have sprouted up like weeds throughout the United States staffed by individuals with little or no formal training. One may look in the Yellow Pages of any telephone book in most communities to find an establishment that will manage chronic pain syndromes including cancer pain. Unfortunately, there are no state regulatory bodies, which govern the way these clinics or physicians practice pain management. Patient influence and persuasion to go to a specific pain clinic is noted in many pain treatment center advertisements, which become unethical if anything is done to interfere with patient free choice through intentional deception or distortion. These abuses are becoming sufficiently common and flagrant.

Patients who are unable to pay are frequently excluded from treatment. If the treatment is as good as advertised in the newspaper, on television or on the radio, why are some patients denied care? The sad fact is that this behavior is legal. Consumer protection legislation and patient education will play an increasingly significant role when one decides to choose a pain treatment center and/or physician. Medical equipment companies in the 1990's also saw the potential to make considerable sums of money by selling devices that could burn nerves, freeze nerves, place salt solutions on nerves or "melt" disc structures in the back. Unfortunately many of these devices have no scientific merit. Medical instrument companies also manufactured electric catheters to be placed in the backs of patients that were intended to diminish pain. There may be medical evidence that these devices diminish pain in a number of select patients with specific pathological entities. This device did provide significant pain relief and did increase the quality of life in many cancer patients. This company then used their technology to provide pain relief in noncancerous pain patients. Unfortunately, they and the other companies required no training by physicians for the implantation of any of these devices. Outside of the medical field, this activity would attract widespread media attention.

Most medical specialties other than pain management require extra training (usually a minimum of 12 months) in a subspecialty of medical training before a physician may refer to themselves as a specialist. However, in pain medicine if an individual is not trained in a procedure the sales representative will come into the operating room (usually without a patient's consent) and instruct a physician on how to do a potentially dangerous procedure or a physician may go to a weekend course sponsored by the manufacturer and practice on a cadaver and subsequently be "certified" as an expert in the performance of a procedure. You should be aware that pharmaceutical representatives may have access to the prescribing habits of physicians. Physicians are frequently enticed into prescribing a certain medication with luncheons, dinners and lavish trips provided by a pharmaceutical company. This practice has been recently documented on a television news story. You should be aware that many of these medications are not safer, better or cheaper than existing medicines.

You should also be aware that the American Board of Medical Specialties has a list of specialties recognized as true medical specialties or subspecialties in the United States. Pain management itself is not included in this list. However, the American Board of Anesthesiology added qualification in pain medicine is recognized. Physicians other than anesthesiologists such as physical medicine and rehabilitation, neurologists etc. can become board certified. This should tell you "Buyer beware!" Many patients use the Internet to access information regarding pain management. In my practice, less than ten percent of patients obtain medical information from an academic source such as the National Library of Congress from computer sources.

The purpose of this book is to inform you that outstanding pain centers do exist throughout the United States but that the "buyer must beware" mentality must be considered with respect to some "injection mills" staffed by some profit only driven individuals with minimal training. The reader must furthermore, be aware that a small number of pain clinics will prescribe potent narcotic medications until an individual becomes addicted. This behavior is not unlike the drug dealer on the street. At the time of your addiction, you must agree to have expensive injection procedures that must be done biweekly with the threat that they are noncompliant if they refuse injections and will have their narcotic prescriptions discontinued. This practice is called "hookem, stickem, and bootem".

The street drug hustler is incarcerated when caught. Nothing happens to the physician who intentionally causes a patient to become addicted to narcotics. On occasion a state medical board will investigate unscrupulous practices. An unscrupulous physician can legally get by with causing a patient's death or in many instances mutilation. The reader of this book will be aware that there is no rationale to ever having any "series" of injections done unless benefit is noted with each injection. Individuals must be aware that some physicians on occasion will entice a patient to have more than one procedure even if the first procedure was ineffective. Usually the physician will recommend three procedures. If the first procedure was properly done why have two more procedures? Two more procedures will make the physician's house payment but probably will not have any effect on your chronic pain. Small pain centers, which have few patients, will entice patients to have three or more injections in a weekly or biweekly series only to increase facility and physician revenues. You will need to learn to distinguish the physician who practices science-based medicine from the physician who is a charlatan.

After completing this book, you should be able to discern what modalities can benefit you and which modalities benefit only the physician. This book may save the person who is suffering from chronic pain, significant time and money by learning what modalities can actually help an individual suffering from chronic pain. If a nerve block is done in the physician's office there is no facility charge. This will save you a facility co-payment. A simplistic approach to successful pain management is to determine the input of a patient's pain and to then end the source of the pain. Imagine a biologic computer mouse continually sending pain impulses to you brain for processing. Decrease the pain signal input by some means and one's pain will decrease.

This book will enable you to gain a basic knowledge of the pathophysiology (the cause of your pain) and treatment of various chronic pain entities. This will enable you to become a team member with your doctor. This knowledge should help prevent you from becoming a potential victim by avoiding the incompetence of certain physicians who claim to be "pain medicine specialists" and by avoiding procedures that are possibly dangerous or have absolutely no scientific merit. This book is written for the layperson suffering from chronic pain. It is hoped that you will derive an understanding of various painful conditions that may affect you or a family member and to relate to you what potentially effective treatments are available to you. You must not become a victim of medical fraud!

# 4. PAIN RELIEF

The ability to relieve pain is very variable and unpredictable, depending on the source or location of pain and whether it is acute or chronic. Pain mechanisms are complex and have peripheral and central nervous system aspects. Therapies should be tailored to the specifics of the pain process or processes in the individual patient. From a computer model, the goal of pain treatment is to decrease electoral input (nerve input) to your brain. Anesthesiologists do nerve blocks and prescribe narcotic medications. Physical medicine and rehabilitation specialists prescribe physical therapy exercises and modalities using heat and cold to relieve pain. Neurologists control pain with anti-seizure medications. Psychiatrists decrease pain with antidepressant drugs. Psychologists manage pain with psychological counseling, hypnosis and biofeedback. Rheumatologists administer steroids into painful joints.

Physical therapists will rehabilitate your body. Chiropractors manipulate your spine to control your back and neck pain by realigning your spine and taking pressure off your nerves. Surgeons operate on nerves, joints and discs to lessen the suffering of pain. In many chronic pain states a multidisciplinary approach using all or most of the mentioned pain specialists is used to manage complex pain problems such as reflex sympathetic dystrophy which will be described in a later chapter. Which modalities actually work? Each of these modalities can help you with your pain. In many instances a multidisciplinary pain center can provide you with the most benefit. You should investigate what therapies are scientifically sound. You should have some basic knowledge about scientific studies that have been.

Suppose your neighbor tells you that you need procedure "X" to manage your pain. Her doctor does this procedure and your neighbor says that her doctor will do it on you. You should take the time to examine studies that recommend this procedure as being wonderful and revolutionary. For example injection "X" is reported in a newspaper advertisement to relieve low back pain in 80% of patients. WOW! This must be a great procedure. You do some investigating. The results are placed in the following table.

| Pain Relief (%) | No Pain Relief (%) |
| --- | --- |

Group I (100 patients) 80 %   20 %
Table 1. Pain relief with new pain device.

What is missing? You need to know how many individuals with the same pain symptoms who did not have this procedure had relief of their pain. On the other hand, you could look at a group of patients with the same treatment who received another drug or substance. This is called a control group. Now compare injection "X" treatment with what is referred to as a sham treatment or a control treatment. . A sham treatment is essentially a placebo treatment. Now examine the results comparing injection "X" with the placebo. The placebo is essentially better than injection "X". A good study will always have a comparison group. Do not be fooled by testimonials or by studies that have no comparison group. Remember that statistics can be manipulated if there is no control group.

|  | Pain Relief (%) | No Pain Relief (%) |
|---|---|---|
| Group I (100 patients) | 80 % | 20 % |
| Group II (100 patients) | 81 % | 19 % |

Table 2. The natural course of the pain is similar to injection X.

You can see now that there is no difference in the groups that received the treatment compared to individuals who did not receive the treatment. You should not be fooled by claims of success that have no merit.

Nerve blocks are frequently used to manage pain. Local anesthetics like Novocain used in combination with steroids are deposited near the nerves or tissues that are responsible for chronic pain. These anesthetics stop pain production by numbing the nerves responsible for your pain. The steroids decrease the irritability of the pain producing nerves. In many instances these blocks will break the pain cycle. Many patients respond to drug therapy. Mild and strong narcotics are prescribed depending on the severity of your pain. Pain patches with either a local anesthetic or a strong narcotic exist which give a patient sustained pain relief. Long acting narcotics (Oxycontin) exist which decrease the need for frequent drug dosing.

Antidepressants and anticonvulsants modulate pain transmission in the spinal cord. Muscle relaxants decrease muscle spasm that can significantly decrease your pain. Non-steroidal anti-inflammatory drugs alleviate pain by decreasing tissue inflammation. The Chinese have used acupuncture for over 2000 years. This method of pain relief consists of placing small needles into the skin and muscles over the body. The needles stimulate larger nerves that go to the spinal cord and release endorphins and enkephalins. These substances decrease the number of pain impulses that go to the brain. Chiropractic therapy consists of manipulating the spine by a physician trained in safe spinal manipulation.

A chiropractor aligns the spine. This maneuver takes pressure off the nerves coming off the spinal cord that decreases pain conduction. Psychologists may help control pain with hypnosis or biofeedback. Hypnosis helps activate the nerves in the spinal cord that block pain signals from traveling up your spinal cord to your brain. Biofeedback uses a machine to enable a pain patient to relax painful muscle. Physical therapists administer modalities that provide heat and cold to your muscles and ligaments. Some therapists do massage therapy that relaxes painful muscles. Electrical stimulation applied to the body decreases pain in a variety of painful conditions. The device is called a TENS (Transcutaneous Electrical Nerve Stimulator) unit. This instrument is battery powered.

A TENS unit stimulates endorphin and enkephalin production in your spinal cord. These devices decrease electrical pain impulses to your brain pain processing section. Neurosurgeons can place implantable devices in your body to control severe pain. One device is called a narcotic pump. This device gives a drop of morphine or other strong narcotic into the fluid around the spinal cord. The other surgically implanted device is called a spinal dorsal column stimulator. A wire is attached to a battery source that is placed in your body. The wire is placed parallel to your spinal cord. This stimulation releases endorphins and enkephalins within the spinal cord. As one can see many modalities are available to patients for the control of their chronic pain. Which one is right for you? The proper treatment for your pain will depend on the severity of your pain as well as your physical and mental health status.

When considering a modality to relieve your pain, you should be aware of another important concept. Evidence-based medicine (EBM) is an attempt to more uniformly apply the standards of evidence gained from scientific medical studies to certain aspects of medical practice. Specifically, EBM seeks to assess the quality of medical evidence relevant to the risks and benefits of treatments (including lack of treatment). According to the Centre for Evidence-Based Medicine, "Evidence-based medicine is the conscientious, explicit and judicious use of current best evidence in making decisions about the care of individual patients. EBM, however, seeks to clarify those parts of medical practice that are in principle subject to scientific methods and to apply these methods to ensure the best prediction of outcomes in medical treatment, even as debate about which outcomes are desirable continues". EBM requires clinical expertise, but also expertise in retrieving, interpreting, and applying the results of scientific studies and in communicating the risks and benefits of different courses of action to patients.

Evidence-based medicine/healthcare is looked upon as a new paradigm, replacing the traditional medical paradigm that is based on standard of care authority (which is common practice in your state). It is dependent on the use of randomized controlled trials, as well as systematic reviews (of a series of trials) and meta-analysis, although it is not restricted to these. There is also an emphasis on the dissemination of information, as well as its collection, so that the evidence can reach clinical practice. It therefore has commonality with the idea of research-based practice.

Having considered the extent to which EBM represents a departure from basing medical decisions on customary practices, there may be a change in the extent to which medical custom remains prevalent in the legal standard of care analysis. A problem ensues in the custom-based standard of care that courts have traditionally used to determine medical malpractice liability. If you are injured from a medical procedure, should the court use the old procedure as the standard of care or the new procedure that is supported by evidence based medicine? For these reasons, current standard of care analysis is potentially inconsistent with the practice of EBM.

This concept is important because traditionally, local customs established the standard of care in medical malpractice actions. Under a custom-based standard, practicing in accordance with accepted practice generally decreases medical liability. Physicians have in the past needed only to conform to the "customs of their peers." As you can see, EBM can cause some legal problems if you are injured from a procedure in a certain medical community. If the standard of care was to do unsafe medicine that EBM demonstrated to be unsafe you need a legal consultation. For example, it used to be acceptable to put steroids in your spinal fluid for the management of back pain. It is no longer the standard of care in most communities. What is your recourse if you had this procedure and developed complications? Complications could take months to years to develop in some instances. You need to realize that EBM practices may differ from customary care in your community

# 5. PAIN DIAGNOSIS

Computers should be evaluated for performance periodically and this concept applies to our bodies. This chapter describes the various diagnostic tests, which may be ordered by your physician. These tests should be ordered to confirm a doctor's clinical impression. Laboratory tests check a sample of your blood, urine or body tissues. Your doctor analyzes the test samples to see if your test results fall within a normal range. The tests use a range because what is normal differs from person to person. Some laboratory tests are precise, reliable indicators of specific health problems. Others provide more general information that simply gives doctors clues to possible health problems. Information obtained from laboratory tests may help doctors decide whether other tests or procedures are needed to make a diagnosis. The information may also help your doctor develop or revise a patient's treatment plan.

All laboratory tests are generally used along with other exams or test such as MRIs, X-rays, EMGs etc. The doctor who is familiar with their patient's medical history and current condition is in the best position to order and to explain test results and their implications. Patients are encouraged to discuss questions or concerns about laboratory test results with the doctor. Two common tests that you should be familiar with are the complete blood count and the blood chemistry tests. A complete blood count measures the levels of different types of blood cells. By determining if there are too many or not enough of each blood cell type, a CBC can help to detect a wide variety of illnesses or signs of infection. A blood chemistry test measures the levels of certain electrolytes, such as sodium and potassium, in your blood. A C reactive protein and erythrocyte sedimentation rate teat may be useful in the diagnosis of rheumatoid arthritis or other inflammatory disease.

Doctors order urine tests to make sure that your kidneys are functioning properly or when they suspect an infection in your kidneys or bladder. This is important if you are taking a medication like a nonsteroidal anti-inflammatory medication that can affect your kidney. A urine test can be done in the doctor's office or even at home. It's easy for toilet-trained kids to give a urine sample since they can urinate in a cup. In other cases a catheter (a narrow, soft tube) can be inserted through the urinary tract opening into the bladder to get the urine sample. Tylenol (acetaminophen) can cause liver damage if you take too much (more than 4000 mg per day). Liver function tests ascertain how your liver is working and helps diagnose any sort liver damage or inflammation. Your doctor may order one when looking for signs of a viral infection or liver damage from other health problems. On occasion, blood tests may be done to determine that you do not have a bleeding problem such as hemophilia. Aspirin can cause bleeding by decreasing the ability of your blood to clot. Before doing a nerve block it is prudent to know if your blood will clot in a normal time. Otherwise a needle can result in significant bleeding.

Plain X rays can be done in a physician's office. X rays can assess bone-joint arthritis. X rays can diagnose degeneration of your discs. Your bone alignment (do the bones line up with each other?) can be assessed as well. Bone fractures can also be identified. You should be aware that you are subject to radiation exposure with this diagnostic test. If you have the possibility of having osteoporosis, your physician may order a DEXA (dual energy x-ray absorptiometry) that is a specific test for the diagnosis of osteoporosis. A Computed Tomography (CT scan) allows a physician to assess a disc in your back as well as arthritic changes affecting the bones in your neck and back. A CT scan of your head can be useful for the diagnosis of a bleeding injury to your brain following trauma to your head. Patients receive radiation exposure with this test. Myelography or a myelogram is primarily of use when surgical therapy is planned. A dye is placed in the fluid that surrounds your spinal cord. An image is formed which tells a physician that a nerve coming off your spinal cord is compressed or not compressed by a disc herniation.

An image does identify painful areas of your body. An image demonstrates abnormal anatomy that could be an area of pain generation. Degenerative disc disease noted on an X-ray for example does not imply that you have a disease or are supposed to have pain. This entity is a normal aspect of aging. Therefore, you should not be alarmed if your doctor tells you that you have degenerative disc disease. The same is true if you are told that you have a disc herniation. Not every disc herniation causes pain and not every disc herniation requires surgery.

Ultrasound is another valuable diagnostic tool. Though ultrasound tests are typically associated with pregnancy, doctors order ultrasounds for different reasons. For example, an ultrasound test can be used to look for collections of fluid in your body, or for problems with your kidneys. An ultrasound is painless and uses high-frequency sound waves to bounce off organs and create a picture. A special jelly is applied to the skin, and a handheld device is moved over the skin. The sound waves that come back produce an image on a screen. Computerized axial tomography is a specialized x ray. CAT scans are a kind of X-ray, and typically are ordered to examine for pathologies such as appendicitis, internal bleeding, or abnormal organ growths. Tomography in which computer analysis of a series of cross-sectional scans made along a single axis of a bodily structure or tissue is used to construct a three-dimensional image of that structure. The technique is used in diagnostic studies of internal bodily structures, as in the detection of tumors or brain aneurysms. A scan is not painful.

A scan may require the use of a contrast material (a dye or other substance) to improve the visibility of certain tissues or blood vessels. The contrast material may be swallowed or given through an IV. CAT scans consist of a highly sensitive x-ray beam that is focused on a specific plane of your body. As this beam passes through your body, it is identified by a detector, which feeds the information that it receives into a computer. The computer then analyzes the information on the basis of tissue density. Generally a CT is preferred where bone details necessary (long bones like your arm or leg, spine, skull), while a MRI produces much better soft tissue details (brain, spinal cord etc.) CT scans are useful for examining body cavities (thorax, abdomen, pelvis) for calcium deposits, cysts, and abscesses.

With some diseases, either a CT scan or MRI is commonly ordered. Spinal stenosis, for example which is a bone growth around your spinal cord or around the holes in the bones of the low back and neck where the nerves from the spinal cord exit to your extremities and is usually seen in individuals over 50 years old. Stenosis can compress the nerves resulting in pain and numbness in the extremities. Because of numbness on the bottom of your feet, you may have difficulty with balance. A CT scan or MRI can identify this pathology. Magnetic Resonance Imaging (MRI) is done by utilization of a magnetic field that is applied around your body. MRIs use radio waves and magnetic fields to produce an image.

MRI's are often used to look at bones, joints, and the brain. Contrast material is sometimes given through an IV in order to get a better picture of certain structures. Nuclei within your body cells with an odd number of protons orient themselves with the magnetic field. The MRI scanner applies a certain amount of energy and the nuclei assume a new orientation with respect to the magnetic field. This energy is removed and the nuclei emit energy as they reorient in the magnetic field. The energy emitted is detected and displayed as an image. The MRI involves no radiation. Magnetic resonance imaging provides a picture of your soft tissue that may be better than the CT scan. A MRI cannot be done if you have certain metals in your body or a heart pacemaker or a defibrillator. Magnetic resonance imaging allows visualization of the discs, spinal cord and cerebrospinal fluid. A MRI can be used with a contrast dye to identify an extruded disc, infection or tumor.

Plain x rays give physicians images in a front to back plane. A side-to-side plane and an oblique view are helpful in diagnosing your possible causes of your pain. On the other hand, a CT and MRI image shows slices of the body as well as a three hundred and sixty degree image of a defined section of the body. Images only show pathology. They do not show pain. Pain is a subjective experience. If you view a photograph of an old scratched and dented computer, you have no idea if it is working or not. You have no idea if it works. The same is true with an X- ray image. An abnormal X ray does not mean that you hurt.

Bone scanning is done using a technetium isotope tracer injected into a vein. This tracer is distributed according to the bone blood flow. A greater blood flow to the bone from trauma such as a fracture or arthritis is compatible with greater bone absorption of the tracer. Total body radiation occurs but is low following a bone scan. The three-phase bone scan consists of the administration of a radioactive tracer followed by scanned images on three occasions. The first image is phase 1 Phase one measures blood flow on the first pass of the tracer. The second phase assesses the blood vessel system while the third phase assesses the turnover of bone, which can be seen in fractures or tumors. Bone scans are frequently used to diagnose RSD.

Electromyography (EMG) and the Nerve Conduction Velocity Tests (NCV) are two diagnostic tools that are helpful to the pain management doctor. These two tests allow the assessment of the location, the pathogenesis, and the prognosis of neuromuscular lesions.

Loss of the outside wrapper (myelin) of a nerve or nerves is assessed by the nerve conduction velocity test. Abnormalities of a nerve take 3-5 days to develop. An EMG is a needle test to determine if your muscle is diseased or injured.

Abnormalities in your muscle can take five to six weeks to become evident. Muscles that are closer to your brain manifest electrophysiological abnormalities sooner than more distal muscles. Focal defects in your nerve may cause NCV slowing across the defect. A NCV measures how fast your nerve sends and impulse. Stimulation of the nerve is done at one end of your nerve and the velocity is measured at another end of your nerve. Generalized nerve pathology results in a reduced nerve conduction velocity. In other words your nerve impulses are slower than normal.

Electromyography (EMG) measures the response of muscles and nerves to electrical activity. It's used to help determine muscle conditions that might be causing muscle weakness, including muscular dystrophy and nerve disorders. A needle electrode is inserted into your muscle (the insertion might feel similar to a pinch) and the signal from the muscle is transmitted from the electrode through a wire to a receiver/amplifier, which is connected to a device that displays readout. EMGs can be uncomfortable and scary to kids, but aren't usually painful. Occasionally kids are sedated while they're done.

Distal latency is the assessment of the distal conduction velocity of your painful nerve that can be affected by the neuromuscular junction that is the location where the nerve and muscle join. Some muscle diseases may have normal NCV studies but electromyographic (EMG) abnormalities usually occur in these situations. EMG measures muscle electrical activity. A reduction in the size of the waves on an oscillo-scope (a screen with waves that move across the screen) is proportional to the nerve loss to the muscle. It should be noted when a muscle is penetrated by an EMG needle, the normal muscle is quiet when it is at rest.

Muscle fiber firing at the time of needle insertion can give your doctor an indication of any muscle disease. The NCV assesses the speed at which your peripheral nerves transmit electrical signals. Your nerve is stimulated, usually with surface electrodes, which are patch-like electrodes placed on your skin over the nerve at various locations. One electrode stimulates the nerve with a very mild electrical impulse. The other electrode records the resulting electrical activity. The distance between electrodes and the time it takes for electrical impulses to travel between electrodes are used to calculate the nerve conduction velocity.

A muscle should contract when stimulated by a nerve impulse. A needle electrode is inserted through the skin into your muscle. There should be a short burst of electrical activity at this time. The electrical activity detected by this electrode is displayed on an oscilloscope, and may be heard through a speaker. After placement of the electrodes, you may be asked to contract certain muscles. The presence, size, and shape of the waveform make up an action potential. This waveform provides information about the ability of your muscle to respond to electrical stimulation. These tests are useful for investigating nerve and muscle function in diseases such as peripheral neuropathy, compression neuropathy etc.

# 6. PAIN DOCTORS

Anyone can work on your computer with no formal training. The same is true with pain management. Did you know that the doctor doing your injection may have trained at a weekend course or may have learned on the job? The weekend courses are cadaver courses. Do you want to be that doctor's first patient? You might be. There are no regulations on pain injectionists. Doctors who manage pain are frequently anesthesiologists. Anesthesiologists ensure that you are safe, pain-free and comfortable during and immediately following surgery. But not everyone realizes that decades of research and work done by anesthesiologists have led to the development of newer, more effective treatments for patients who have pain unrelated to surgery. Many techniques used to make surgery and childbirth virtually painless is now being used to relieve other types of pain. In fact, the work pioneered by anesthesiologists has led to treatments for pain control outside the operating room.

Frequently an anesthesiologist heads a team of other specialists and doctors who work together to help you manage your pain. Pain medicine doctors are supposed to be experts at diagnosing why you are having pain as well as treating the pain itself. Some of the more common pain problems they manage include: arthritis, back and neck pain, cancer pain, nerve pain, migraine headaches, shingles, phantom limb pain for amputees and pain caused by AIDS. Pain medicine doctors are experts at diagnosing why you are having pain as well as treating your pain.

Like other physicians, anesthesiologists have completed four years of medical school. They spent four more years learning anesthesiology and pain medicine during residency training. Many anesthesiologists who specialize in pain medicine receive an additional year of fellow-ship training to become an expert in treating pain. Some also have done research, and many have special certification in pain medicine through the American Board of Anesthesiology. This board is the only organization recognized by the American Board of Medical Specialties to offer special credentials in pain medicine. Medical specialty certification in the United States is a voluntary process. While medical licensure sets the minimum competency requirements to diagnose and treat patients, it is not specialty specific. Board certification demonstrates a physician's expertise in a particular specialty and/or subspecialty of medical practice. Pain medicine is a subspecialty of anesthesiology.

The American Board of Medical Specialties member boards (24) are responsible for setting the standards for quality practice in a particular medical specialty. Each Member Board has a board of trustees or directors, all of whom are certified in that Board's medical specialty. Individual Member Boards evaluate physician candidates to ascertain if the candidate completed the appropriate residency requirements and if he or she has an institutional or valid license to practice medicine. If a physician meets these basic admission standards, the Member Board will evaluate the candidate using written and oral examinations. Because specialties differ so widely, the criteria that inform these tests are quite different. What makes someone a good anesthesiologist does not necessarily make him or her a competent cardiologist.

Ultimately, the measure of physician specialists is not merely that they have been certified, but that they keep current in their specialty. The American Board of Medical Specialties requires maintenance of certification that is a formal means of measuring a physician's continued competency in his or her certified specialty and/or subspecialty. To become recertified a physician must: hold a valid, unrestricted medical license, meet educational and self-assessment programs determined by the particular Board, demonstrate specialty-specific skills and knowledge, demonstrate the use of best evidence and practices compared to peers and national benchmarks.

Unfortunately, in many states a physician needs no credentials to practice pain management other than a medical or osteopathic medicine degree and a state medical license. As a result, there are no guidelines as to who can call themselves a pain medicine "specialist". There are no local, state or national standards with respect to pain management. The American Academy of Pain Medicine, the American Academy of Pain Management, and the American Board of Anesthesiologists administer written examinations to certify pain management doctors. These organizations provide continuing education courses annually. Some physicians do not certify through one of these organizations but classify themselves as pain physicians. They may go to a weekend cadaver course to be able to do a certain procedure. You should ascertain that you are not the first live patient that one of these doctors practices on after finishing a weekend cadaver course. Other professionals (plumbers, nurses, teachers, policemen, etc.) must have formal training to practice their profession. Pain doctors in many instances do not! Does this frighten you? It should!! I recommend that you investigate your prospective pain physician before you receive treatments that will not benefit you or may actually harm you.

Ask to see your physician's credentials. Hospitals in many instances may want anyone who will show up and has a medical degree to do potentially mutilating procedures on patients who have insurance. You should ascertain if your pain doctor has completed a fellowship (specialized training in pain medicine) or has sufficient experience through residency training to do a procedure on you. With these facts in mind, you must do your homework when choosing a pain medicine physician. Most university pain centers require that pain medicine physicians have a formal fellowship before they can begin to treat patients.

Be aware that some pain physicians are unable to be certified in any specialty. They may then call themselves "pain specialists" and begin harming patients. It is your duty to find the best-trained physician. Your insurance plan will list doctors approved by their plan. Some companies have strict criteria before admitting physicians to their plan. The American Association of health plans lists a Web site with a doctor finder at www.aahp.org. Click on to this site and follow the instructions to help locate a physician. A background information check can be done on every physician. Go to ama-assn.org/aps/amahg.htm. Has your physician ever been disciplined by a state medical board? Find out by going to the Web site ama-assn.org/ama/pubcategory/2645.html to find out if your doctor is a health hazard. If your doctor has been disciplined find out the reason.

A physician should have some certification from a medical specialty like anesthesiology, physical medicine etc. to do pain medicine in addition to completion of a fellowship. Ideally, the pain medicine physician should have further training in pain medicine. If your physician has no certification in any specialty you should eliminate that physician from your list of potential treating physicians. There may be some qualified doctors who have not taken a certification test but it would be extremely difficult identifying those individuals who are truly competent. You should ask your physician if he or she has credentials in pain medicine including research publications etc. To ascertain if your physician is certified by the American Board of Medical Specialties, go to the website www.ABMS.org.

# 7. OPIOID MEDICATIONS

Powerful drugs affect the brain as well as nerves throughout your body. The "human computer" CPU is affected, and pain impulses from your body are slowed down as well as the spinal cord pain intensity transmission. Narcotic drugs are prescribed for postoperative pain, cancer pain and for some chronic pain syndromes. Narcotic drugs can relieve moderate to severe pain. The term narcotic refers to agents that benumb or deaden nerves, causing loss of feeling or paralysis. Psychedelic drugs like LSD, contrary to popular belief are not narcotics. Many law enforcement officials in the United States inaccurately use the word "narcotic" to refer to any illegal drug or any unlawfully possessed drug. The Federal government is attempting to decrease the use of these chemicals because of the addictive and abuse potentials. Most medical professionals prefer the term opioid which refers to natural, semi-synthetic and synthetic substances that behave pharmacologically like morphine. The Opioids are a class of controlled pain-management drugs that contain natural or synthetic chemicals based on morphine, the active component of opium. These narcotics effectively mimic the pain-relieving chemicals that the body produces naturally. Opioids are the most often prescribed pain-relievers because they are so effective.

Morphine is the standard to which other opioid drugs are compared. Morphine is frequently prescribed to alleviate severe pain after surgery. Codeine can be helpful in soothing somewhat milder pain, as are oxycodone (OxyContin, an oral, controlled-release form of the drug), propoxyphene (Darvon), hydrocodone (Vicodin), hydromorphone (Dilaudid) and meperidine (Demerol), which is used less often because of its side effects. Diphenoxylate or Lomotil can also relieve severe diarrhea, and codeine can ease severe coughs.

The primary medical use of opioids is to relieve pain. Other medical uses include control of coughs and diarrhea, and the treatment of addiction to other opioids. Opioids can produce euphoria, making them prone to abuse. Opioids should only be used for moderate to severe pain that has not responded to non-narcotic drugs like aspirin or ibuprofen. Narcotics can be used alone like oxycodone or used in combination with aspirin, ibuprofen or acetaminophen (Tylenol).

Some narcotics like oxycodone or morphine are available as an extended release tablet that must be swallowed whole. Tablets, which are not extended release, may be split..

In 1914, the Federal Government passed a law that prohibited prescribing opioid drugs for recreational use. The Federal Controlled Sub-stances Act of 1970 formulated schedules for drugs. You need to be aware of three of five schedules; 1. has no current accepted medical use like heroin or marijuana, 2. high abuse and dependence potential like morphine, codeine or oxycodone, and 3. includes drugs with a lesser dependence and abuse liability. Hydrocodone (Vicodin) is a schedule 2 drug. Valium, a relaxant is a schedule III drug and some cough medicines are schedule 4 drugs. Oxycodone (Oxycotin) is a schedule II drug which means that it is potentially more habit forming than Schedule 3 0r 4 drugs.

There is a difference between the descriptions of narcotic drugs and opioids. Opioids are drugs like morphine, hydrocodone etc. Narcotics are extremely addictive drugs and include heroin and other drugs that can cause sedation. Opioids act by attaching to a group of proteins called opioid receptors, found in the brain, spinal cord and gastrointestinal tract. When these drugs link to certain opioid receptors in the brain and spinal cord they can block the transmission of pain messages to the brain.

For the purposes of discussion in outlining the pharmacologic activity of these compounds, the opioids will be classified as (1) agonists, (2) antagonists, and (3) mixed agonist-antagonists. All drugs bind to receptors that exist on the outer membrane of your cells. Narcotics bind to narcotic receptors on cells in the brain and spinal cord. Opioid receptors may also be recruited on tissue cells outside of your central nervous system such as your knee following an injury. An injection of morphine into your knee may alleviate your pain.

When opioids turn on a receptor, that receptor decreases pain signals usually in your spinal cord that prevents pain signals from going to your brain. As a result, your pain perception is decreased. Experimental studies involving binding of opioids to specific receptors in the brain and spinal cord have substantiated the hypothesis that these receptors exist which mediates the actions of the opioid drugs to stop pain signals to your brain. There are two basic classes of opioid receptors called mu and kappa receptors. Other classes exist (e.g. delta) but are not important for the discussion of your pain in this chapter. These receptors also appear to be the site of action of the endogenous (pain drugs produced by your body) opioid-like substances and have been divided into three major categories, designated mu, and kappa.

It has also been proposed that at least two subtypes of each category of opioid receptors exist. Experimental evidence suggests that activation of mu receptors (found principally at sites in the brain) is associated with analgesia, respiratory depression, euphoria, and physical dependence. The kappa receptors (located within the spinal cord) are believed to mediate spinal analgesia, constriction of the pupil size and sedation. The other receptors may influence affective behavior, and although some physicians believe that activation of these receptors plays a role in opioid-induced analgesia, this remains controversial.

Since a number of different compounds, (e.g., certain antihistamines, some steroids, and anti-psychotics have phencyclidine) none of which are opioid in structure but can affect binding affinity for these sites. Agonistic (stimulating) opioids act as analgesics by binding to and activating both mu and kappa receptors in the brain and spinal cord. The opioid antagonists bind to all categories of opioid receptor sites throughout the body, but fail to activate them. These compounds are not used for pain control; rather, the utility of these drugs lies in their ability to reverse an overdose of opioids including narcotics.

The compounds that comprise the mixed agonist-antagonist group are more recent additions to the clinically important opioids. These drugs are semi-synthetic derivatives of morphine, the chemical structures of which have agonistic activity at some kappa receptors but antagonistic activity at mu receptors, e.g., pentazocine, butorphanol, and nalbu-phine, or partial agonistic activity at mu receptors and antagonistic activity at kappa receptors, eg. buprenorphine. All are effective analgesics since they stimulate either mu or kappa receptors.

Chemically, the opioid agonists include a number of classes of drugs, all of which have pharmacologic effects similar to those of morphine. Morphine is the oldest known drug of this class. It remains as the prototype for the opioid group and is the standard to which all other opioid analgesic drugs are compared. Opioid drugs decrease pain but also affect all organ systems. Your pituitary gland in your brain can be adversely affected by chronic narcotic use. For example in males opioids can decrease testosterone that can cause depression and erectile dysfunction. Drowsiness and blurred vision can occur. Changes in mood can occur. An inability to concentrate can occur.

Euphoria can be experienced in 20% of individuals taking opioid drugs. Euphoria can be the cause of addiction. Opioids can stop your respiratory drive that can cause you to stop breathing. Narcotics affect your stomach by slowing down the passage of food in combination with your brain to cause nausea and vomiting. Opioids can cause a significant decrease in your blood pressure that may cause you to fall. Opioids decrease movement of the bowel resulting in constipation. Morphine can make gall bladder disease worse by contracting a valve where the gall bladder meets the intestine called the sphincter of Oddi. Opioid drugs can result in a release of histamine from certain cell in the body that can cause itching and a rash. As you can see opioid drugs can have side effects.

Tolerance, addiction and physical dependence can occur with opioid drugs. Tolerance occurs when it takes more of the drug to cause the same decrease in your pain. This is not addiction. Patients may find that they develop tolerance to opioid pain medications and may need to have their doses increased in order to be effective. Tolerance has not been shown to lead to drug addiction. Physical dependence is a condition that occurs when continued use of the drug is needed to prevent a withdrawal reaction. Steady use of opioids can result in tolerance to the drugs so that higher doses must be taken to achieve the same effects. Long-term use also can lead to physical dependence—the body adapts to the presence of the drug and withdrawal symptoms occur if use is reduced abruptly.

Addiction is an intense craving for an opioid and is often associated with recreational use. Signs and symptoms of addiction include yawning, sweating, restlessness, irritability, anxiety, nasal discharge, tearing, dilated pupils, gooseflesh, tremors, loss of appetite, body aches, nausea and vomiting, fever and chills and an increase in heart rate and blood pressure. These symptoms last approximately 7-10 days. Minor symptoms can begin in 8-12 hours after the last dose of the opioid. The more severe symptoms like nausea and vomiting begin 48-72 hours after the last dose of the drug. With respect to agonist drugs, morphine is the prototype. It can be administered by mouth, rectum or by injection into muscle or vein. Is is prepared in a capsule, tablet or a liquid. It is available by a rectal suppository as well. This route of administration is used for those patients who cannot swallow or are having severe vomiting. Hydromorphone and oxymorphone also come in the form of rectal suppositories. The duration of action of opioids varies from drug to drug. Sustained release morphine and oxycodone give a longer duration of action. Immediate release drugs (eg. OXIR) give a faster onset but have a shorter duration of action. Fentanyl, which is 75 times more potent than morphine is available in a patch and sucker, forms. The fentanyl patch is used for severe constant pain. The pain relief is continuous. The sucker, which only comes in a raspberry flavor, is used for severe cancer pain in instances where the severe pain fluctuates. Fentora is another oral form of fentanyl. With respect to the fentanyl pain patch, the amount of drug released is controlled by small holes in a membrane in the patch. A larger hole permits the release of fentanyl into your body. The patches are available in different doses. The fentanyl is released for 48-72 hours. Patients with a fever can be at a risk for an overdose as the amount of fentanyl administered to your body can increase by 25% for every 30C increase in body temperature. The advantage of the patch is that patients do not have to take frequent pills during the night. The patch should be applied to a hairless surface.

Codeine is a weaker medication that is used to treat mild pain. They may be combined with acetaminophen to make each more potent. You need to be aware that smoking tobacco can decrease the potency of Darvon and hydrocodone. Tramadol (Ultram) is an interesting drug and may be used for moderate to moderately severe pain. It has a low abuse potential. It is a scheduled IV drug. It activates mu and kappa receptors. The side effects are minimal when compared to opioid drugs. Tramadol does not produce withdrawal symptoms like opioids.

The advantage of tramadol over other drugs is that tramadol inhibits norepinephrine and serotonin. These two substances in the brain and spinal cord can increase your pain. The opioid drugs do not have this effect. Tramadol can cause nausea dizziness and headaches. Tramadol does not lower the heart rate or blood pressure. Tramadol provides pain relief similar to codeine and propoxyphene. Naloxone and naltrexone are drugs that reverse the respiratory effects of opioids. Naltrexone can be given orally. The only time that these drugs are given is to treat opioid intoxication. Butorphanol (Stadol) is a mixed agonist-antagonists drug. This drug displays receptor selectivity and stimulates kappa receptors. These drugs have less opioid abuse tendencies than the agonist drugs. Opioids on the other hand work on both mu and kappa receptors. Strong opioids exist which are usually reserved for cancer patients or other patients with severe pain.

Hydromorphone (Dilaudid) and levorphanol (Levo-Droman) are eight and five times more potent than morphine. Meperidine (Demerol) is an opioid that is weaker than morphine. It is used infrequently in pain management as it can cause tremors or seizures if used on a chronic basis. Methadone is a synthetic drug similar to morphine. The ad-vantage of methadone for your pain management is that it does not cause euphoria. Methadone however, can cause a conduction problem in your heart. Consequently, patients have died from heart problems after being prescribed methadone. Hydrocodone and oxycodone are two opioids used for moderate to moderately severe pain. These drugs are usually combined with aspirin and acetaminophen which can potentiate the analgesic efficacy of these drugs.

Another fact that you need to know is that opioid drugs can actually cause you to experience increased pain. This observation is called opioid induced pain. Instead of decreasing your biologic CPU it can stimulate pain perception in your brain. Many physicians are unaware of this fact. In this situation, a reduction in your dose of your medicine or stopping it can actually decrease your pain. This phenomenon can also be seen in patents that have spinal morphine drug delivery systems.

As one can see, there are many opioids that can be used for the management of your acute and chronic pain. The proper choice of your medication is dependent upon the magnitude of your pathology, the side effects of the drug prescribed, the effectiveness of the drug and your overall health.

# 8. ADDICTION

Addiction alters your central processing unit and short circuits your brain synapses causing a person to crave more of a chemical substance. Drugs are chemicals that have a profound impact on the neurochemical balance in your brain. This action affects how you feel and act. People who are suffering emotionally use drugs to escape from their problems. This can lead to drug abuse and addiction. Some physicians are afraid to prescribe scheduled drugs because of the possibility of causing addiction. Addiction is a chronic relapsing brain disease. Brain imaging shows that addiction severely alters your brain areas critical to decision-making, learning and memory, and behavior control, which may help to explain the compulsive and destructive behaviors of addiction. An addiction is a recurring problem by an individual to engage in some specific activity, despite harmful consequences to the individual's health, mental state or social life.

An addiction can occur with drugs, gambling, overeating etc. Drugs can make you euphoric. As a result, you may request more and more drugs to maintain this euphoria. Drug abuse or substance abuse, involves the repeated and excessive use of prescription or street drugs. In one way or another, almost all drugs over stimulate the pleasure center of the brain, flooding it with the neurotransmitter dopamine which produces euphoria. That heightened sense of pleasure can be so compelling that the brain wants that feeling back, again and again. Addiction is frequently found in people with a wide variety of mental illnesses, including anxiety disorders, unipolar and bipolar depression, schizophrenia, and borderline and other personality disorders. Methadone can be used for the treatment of pain in addicted patients. Methadone is also an opiate that prevents users from getting high on heroin by competing with the much more potent opiates for the body's opiate receptors. Buprenophrine is another drug that is effective for the treatment of addiction and is also an analgesic.

Addiction and drug dependence occur when drugs become so important that you are willing to sacrifice your work, home and even your family. Once your brain and body get used to the substances you are taking, you begin to require increasingly larger and more frequent doses, in order to achieve the same effect. Narcotics such as Heroin may over-stimulate the pleasure centers of the brain producing euphoric effects that cause compulsive drug-seeking behaviors. The severities of withdrawal symptoms associated with narcotics include chills, shakes, muscle pain, nausea, vomiting, and headaches and cravings.

A clinician must be able to distinguish between legitimate patients with chronic pain and individuals engaged in non-therapeutic drug seeking behavior. Physicians have for years recognized the value of opioid analgesics in relieving chronic pain. Unfortunately, drug seekers may also request opioid analgesics. They do this by feigning illnesses, and seek controlled substances from multiple doctors and by forge prescriptions. Drug seekers may be difficult to distinguish from true chronic pain sufferers. In general, drug seekers prefer illicit drugs such as heroin and cocaine to prescription drugs. Prescription drugs however, have advantages over illicit drugs. Third-party insurers or welfare-entitlement programs may pay for prescribed drugs. Prescription pharmaceuticals are obtained in the safety of the physician's office.

Drug abuse and addiction have a devastating impact on society. Heroin use alone is responsible for the epidemic number of new cases of HIV/AIDS and hepatitis. Drug abuse is responsible for decreased job productivity and attendance, increased healthcare costs, and an escalation of domestic violence and violent crimes.

An estimated 20 percent of people in the United States have used prescription drugs for nonmedical reasons. Central nervous stimulants, depressants and opioids are prescription drugs that are frequently abused. Central nervous system depressants are used to treat anxiety, panic attacks, and sleep disorders. Examples are Nembutal (pentobarbital sodium), Valium (diazepam), and Xanax (alprazolam). Long-term use can lead to physical dependence and addiction. Central nervous system stimulants are used to treat narcolepsy and the attention deficit/hyperactivity disorder. Examples include Ritalin (methylphenidate) and Dexedrine (dextroamphetamine). Opioids, also known as narcotic analgesics are used to treat pain. Opioids are the most commonly abused prescription drugs. Examples include morphine, codeine, OxyContin (oxycodone), Vicodin (hydrocodone) and Demerol (meperidine).

One may obtain drugs by the following means: prescription forgery, by telephone (faking to be a physician's office), multiple doctors, and indiscriminate prescribing by physicians. Pain clinicians who prescribe chronic opioids are aware that there is an illicit market for opioid analgesics. For example Oxycontin can be sold for $1.00 per milligram. One 80 mg pill can be sold on the street for $80.00. Telephone scams occur when the drug seeker claims to be a patient of one of the other physicians in the on-call group, and asks for a prescription for an analgesic to last until they can see their regular physician. Sometimes, the drug seeker uses a telephone to impersonate a practicing physician.

Prescription forgery is a common activity among drug seekers. Drug seekers can modify a legitimate prescription to increase the dosage or quantity of an opioid. The easiest method is to increase the number of tablets on the prescription. Multiple episodes of noncompliance raise an alert of drug seeking behavior as well as multiple episodes of prescription loss. The patient with chemical dependency loses control over drug taking. The patient cannot take medications as prescribed. The patient repeatedly reports lost or stolen medications. The physician will notice that the drug seeker frequently requests early renewals of prescriptions. A pain physician must however, be aware that aggressive complaining about the need for more drugs may indicate inadequate pain management as opposed to drug seeking behavior. A patient should not be allowed to suffer. It should be understood that substance abusers can suffer from chronic pain which should be treated in a humane manner.

Unapproved use of opioids to treat another symptom such as sleep deprivation should not be tolerated. However, the pain management physician must objectively identify a patient's pain complaint with the appropriate medical test before prescribing an opioid. Opioid analgesics are powerful tools in the armamentarium of the pain clinician. Criminal and chemically dependent drug seekers may attempt to obtain such drugs from the physician.

A pain medicine physician must therefore, use safe prescribing strategies. A physician has no legal obligation to prescribe opioid analgesics on demand. A reasonable precaution to be taken by the pain medicine physician with an unfamiliar patient is to establish a policy of not prescribing opioid analgesics pending a complete assessment including corroboration of the patient's history. Some patients or patient families are afraid of addiction. However, a significant number of individuals do not understand the difference between addiction and tolerance.

The American Academy of Pain Medicine, the American Pain Society, and the American Society of Addiction Medicine recognize the following definitions and recommend their use.

I. Addiction: Addiction is a primary, chronic, neurobiological disease, with genetic, psychosocial, and environmental factors influencing its development and manifestations. It is characterized by behaviors that include one or more of the following: impaired control over drug use, compulsive use, continued use despite harm, and craving. An entity termed pseudo-addiction exists which is not true addiction. Pseudo-addiction occurs when pain is under treated. Pseudo addiction resolves when the pain resolves. Addictive behavior on the other hand, persists in spite of increasing the patient's pain medication.

II. Physical Dependence: Physical dependence is a state of adaptation that is manifested by a drug class specific withdrawal syndrome that can be produced by abrupt cessation, rapid dose reduction, decreasing blood level of the drug, and/or administration of an antagonist.

III. Tolerance: Tolerance is a state of adaptation in which exposure to a drug induces changes that result in a diminution of one or more of the drug's effects over time. Most specialists in pain medicine and addiction medicine agree that patients treated with prolonged opioid therapy usually do develop physical dependence and sometimes develop tolerance, but do not usually develop addictive disorders. Addiction is a primary chronic disease and exposure to opioid medications is only one of the etiologic factors in its development. Therefore, good clinical judgment must be used in determining whether the pattern of behaviors signals the presence of addiction or reflects a different issue.

# 9. NON-STEROIDAL MEDICATIONS

Steroids are drugs used to reduce inflammatory pain such as arthritic joint pain. However, steroids may have significant side effects associated with their use. For example, steroids can cause weight gain, osteoporosis, avascular necrosis of your hips etc. Nonsteroidal anti-inflammatory drugs are commonly used to treat painful conditions. This may include a sprain strain injury, a headache, a toothache etc. M any individuals believe that these drugs are safe because many of them are sold over the counter. However, these drugs may have serious side effects in some individuals.

Nonsteroidal anti-inflammatory drugs inhibit prostaglandins. These biochemicals decrease input of pain signals to your brain for central processing. Prostaglandins are a related family of chemicals that are produced by the cells of your body and have several important functions. They promote inflammation, pain, and cause fevers. They are involved with the function of platelets that are necessary for the clotting of your blood, and protect the lining of your stomach from the damaging effects of acid. Prostaglandins are produced within your body's cells by the enzyme cyclooxygenase (COX). There are two of these enzymes, Cox 1 and Cox 2. However, only Cox-1 produces prostaglandins that support platelets and protect the stomach. In essence, these chemicals decrease the pain signals which are sent to your brain's processing area. Nonsteroidal anti-inflammatory drugs (NSAIDs) block the Cox enzymes and reduce prostaglandins throughout your body. As a consequence, ongoing inflammation, pain, and fever are reduced. Since the prostaglandins that protect the stomach and support the platelets and blood clotting also are reduced, NSAIDs can cause ulcers in your stomach and cause bleeding. NSAIDs differ in how strongly they inhibit Cox-1 and, therefore, in their tendency to cause ulcers and promote bleeding.

Another important difference between the two enzymes is their ability to cause ulcers and bleeding. The more an NSAID blocks Cox-1, the greater is its tendency to cause ulcers and bleeding. One NSAID called Celebrex, blocks Cox-2, but has little effect on Cox-1. This drug is referred to as one of the selective Cox-2 inhibitors and therefore causes less bleeding and fewer ulcers than other NSAIDs. Aspirin is the only NSAID that is able to inhibit the clotting of blood for a prolonged period (4 to 7 days). This prolonged effect of aspirin makes it an ideal drug for preventing the blood clots that cause heart attacks and strokes.

COX-2 inhibitors do not cause your blood to not clot. This is one reason why COX-2 inhibitors are implicated in heart attacks. You should be aware that the FDA issued a public health advisory concerning use of non-steroidal anti-inflammatory drug products including those known as COX-2 selective agents. The COX-2 selective agents like Celebrex may be associated with an increased risk of serious cardiovascular events especially when they are used for long periods of time or in very high-risk settings. The drugs Vioxx and Bextra have been taken off the market. Preliminary results from a long-term clinical trial suggest that long-term use of a non-selective NSAID; naproxen may be associated with an increased cardiovascular risk compared to placebo.

The FDA (Federal Drug Administration) stated that patients who are at a high risk of gastrointestinal bleeding, have a history of intolerance to non-selective NSAIDs, or are not doing well on non-selective NSAIDs may be appropriate candidates for COX-2 selective agents. Non-selective NSAIDs are widely used in both over-the-counter and prescription settings. As prescription drugs, many are approved for short-term use in the treatment of pain and menstrual discomfort, and for longer-term use to treat the signs and symptoms of osteoarthritis and rheumatoid arthritis.

NSAIDS are classified as non-opioid analgesic drugs and are aspirin like drugs. Although the pharmacologic and toxicological properties of these compounds are similar and all possess analgesic activity, only certain drugs are indicated specifically for the relief of pain (eg. Feldene, Voltaren, Advil, Naprosyn, Celebrex etc,). NSAIDS stop the production of prostaglandin production. Since prostaglandins are formed and released in response to cell membrane injury, these substances have become associated with pain reactions that accompany tissue injury and inflammation. Prostaglandins sensitize pain receptors (mostly C fibers) by lowering the threshold to thermal, mechanical and chemical stimuli.

Thus, the increased pain sensations induced by prostaglandins is a localized event that allows the mediators of pain such as bradykinin, histamine and substance p, to exert a greater effect on pain receptors. The receptors are stimulated to a greater extent causing more pain. All of the NSAIDS analgesics prevent the biosynthesis and release of prostaglandins by inhibition of prostaglandin cyclooxygenase, a cell membrane enzyme that is present in almost all cells. Therefore, the NSAIDS reduce the formation of prostaglandins and decrease the pain sensitivity caused by these substances. NSAIDS have analgesic, fever reducing, and anti-inflammatory effects.

Not all of the drugs are equally active, nor are all clinically useful, with respect to these effects. Dolobid (diflunisal) for example, is used exclusively as an analgesic but does not decrease a fever. With the exception of acetaminophen, aspirin, and ibuprofen, none of the other compounds are used to reduce fever. NSAIDS are used in the treatment of various arthritic conditions such as rheumatoid arthritis, ankylosing spondylitis, osteoarthritis and acute gouty arthritis. As the particular inflammatory condition being treated is alleviated, the pain associated with the disease is also decreased. Pain associated with inflammatory diseases is effectively reduced by all of these NSAID drugs. Aspirin is the oldest NSAID. Toradol (ketolorac) has minimal antiinflammatory effects but has significant pain relieving effects. This observation suggests that antiinflammatory effects are not related to pain relieving effects. NSAIDS have a ceiling affect. This means that when you take a certain dose of an NSAID, more of the NSAID will not give you more pain relief. This affect is opposite to that of opioid analgesics. They have no ceiling effects. This means that more of an opioid will increase your pain relief.

The Bayer Company in Germany discovered aspirin in the late 1800's. Aspirin is the prototype to which other NSAIDS are compared. The side effects of the NSAIDS should be briefly discussed. Serious side effects are rare. The liver and kidneys can be affected by high doses of NSAIDS prescribed over a long duration. Patients with forms of arthritis will require NSAIDS long term for the anti-inflammatory properties of the NSAIDS.

Gastrointestinal toxicity can occur with all NSAIDS that can lead to bleeding from the stomach and may lead to hospitalization and surgery as well as blood transfusions. Localized irritation of the stomach lining constitutes the most common adverse reaction associated NSAIDS. Although epigastric distress is common at the lower doses, gastric and/or intestinal ulceration and bleeding will occur in only a small percentage of patients. At higher doses of aspirin, erosive gastritis and gastrointestinal hemorrhage is observed more often. These effects are the result of the inhibition of cyclooxygenase 1 (COX-1). You need cyclooxygenase 1 to form protective prostaglandins that reduce acid secretion by your stomach and promote the secretion of protective intestinal mucus. Aspirin and other compounds with high anti-inflammatory activity, such as indomethacin, tend to elicit the highest incidence of gastrointestinal reactions. Other NSAIDS like naproxen are considered to produce fewer and less intense gastrointestinal reactions than aspirin.

Acetaminophen is essentially devoid of these effects. Acetaminophen has some anti-inflammatory affects. Newer NSAIDS that are specific for cyclo-oxygenase 2 enzymes are safer than the rest of the NSAIDS that inhibit both cyclooxygenase 1 and 2. Celebrex is safer on your stomach. With respect to the heart and lungs all of the NSAIDS can cause swelling in your extremities as well as increase your blood pressure. It should be noted that all NSAIDS including ibuprofen and naproxen could be linked to an increased risk of a heart attack. Because of this research, it is advisable to use the lowest effective dose of NSAID for the shortest time necessary, NSAIDS can cause clotting problems and make you prone to bleeding or bruising. This is due to the inhibition of thromboxane A, formation in thrombocytes (cells in the bloodstream associated with clotting). However, Celebrex does not cause this problem. In other words, Celebrex is the only NSAID that does not adversely affect the blood thinning effects of aspirin.

With respect to your kidneys, sodium and water retention with extremity swelling are seen with NSAID use. The higher the dose, the more prone you are for these side effects. Ask your doctor about the lowest effective dose that can be prescribed for you. If you are over sixty years of age you should be prescribed lower doses, as you may be more sensitive to NSAIDS than younger patients. NSAIDS are excellent analgesic medications for pain in extremities, as well as for dental pain and headaches. They are furthermore, non-addicting. NSAIDS should be used with caution in elderly patients. If you are significantly sick (such as an intensive care patient, an NSAID can adversely affect your kidneys. In some instances NSAIDS can cause kidney failure.

Nonsteroidal anti-inflammatory drugs (NSAIDs) are commonly used in the elderly for the treatment of fever, pain, pain associated with inflammation in rheumatoid arthritis and osteoarthritis, neuromuscular disorders, headache, and musculoskeletal conditions. Each year in the United States, people spend 5 to 10 billion dollars to purchase prescription and over-the-counter NSAIDs. Gastrointestinal side effects such as ulcers and bleeding are the most prevalent and life-threatening problems associated with NSAIDs in elderly individuals.

Specifically in the elderly, NSAIDs have become a leading cause of hospitalization in this age group and may increase the risk of death from ulceration more than four fold. NSAIDs and the new class of cyclo-oxygenase-2 selective NSAIDs continue as drugs of choice for analgesia and anti-inflammatory effects. Physiological changes of aging worsen the side-effect profile of NSAIDs in the elderly. These side effects, when added to the increased potential for drug interactions, lead to a much greater risk for adverse outcomes when NSAIDs are used in the elderly patient.

NSAIDS should be used with caution in pregnant patients as well. These drugs are not recommended during pregnancy, especially in the third trimester. While NSAIDs as a class are not direct congenital malformation drugs. They may however, cause premature closure of the fetal ductus arteriosus and also cause a reduction in maternal amniotic fluid. As a result, pregnant patients taking NSAIDS may require ultrasound monitoring by the treating obstetrician. In addition NSAIDS may cause premature birth. Aspirin should not be used during pregnancy. Fetal bleeding could occur as a result of the inhibitory effects on the fetal platelets. Acetaminophen which does have slight anti-inflammatory properties is safe and well-tolerated during pregnancy.

# 10. MUSCLE RELAXANTS

Muscle relaxants are effective for short-term symptomatic relief in patients with acute and chronic low back pain. However, the incidence of drowsiness, dizziness and other side effects is high. Muscle relaxants must be used with caution. Muscle relaxants are a useful adjunct in the treatment of patients with chronic and persistent pain. There are a number of categories in muscle relaxants, but one may broadly divide them into centrally acting muscle relaxants and peripherally acting muscle relaxants. Central mechanisms of action include activity on the glycine receptors, as seen with the muscle relaxant properties of benzodiazepines, or on the GABA receptors, as seen with benzodiazepines and baclofen. Baclofen has been used to treat the spasticity of multiple sclerosis; it may also be used to treat muscle spasm associated with radiculopathy. Cyclobenzaprine differs from amitriptyline by two hydrogen ions, and it retains many of the side effects of amitriptyline (e.g., dry mouth, constipation, irregular heartbeats). Data transmission is the process of sending digital or analog data over a communication medium to one or more computing, network, communication or electronic devices. It enables the transfer and communication of devices in a point-to-point, point-to-multipoint and multipoint-to-multipoint environment. Like a computer, muscle relaxants decrease signals from your body's peripheral system to the spinal cord.

Muscle relaxants are effective for short-term symptomatic relief in patients with acute and chronic low back pain. However, the incidence of drowsiness, dizziness and other side effects is high. Muscle relaxants must be used with caution. Muscle relaxants are a useful adjunct in the treatment of patients with chronic and persistent pain. There are a number of categories in muscle relaxants, but one may broadly divide them into (1) centrally acting muscle relaxants and (2) peripherally acting muscle relaxants. If your muscles are tense, you can have decreased oxygen in your muscle tissue that can cause you to experience pain. Muscle relaxants are drugs that decrease tension in your muscles. These drugs can be useful in pain management. Muscle relaxants are not really a single class of drugs, but are a group of different drugs and each of these drugs can have an overall sedative effect on your body. These drugs other than dantrolene do not act directly on your muscles, but they act in your brain and are more of a total body relaxant.

Skeletal muscle relaxants are drugs that relax striated muscles (those that control your skeleton). Skeletal muscle relaxants may be used for relief of spasticity in neuromuscular diseases, such as multiple sclerosis, as well as for spinal cord injury and stroke. They may also be used for pain relief in minor strain injuries and control of the muscle symptoms of tetanus. The muscle relaxants may be divided into only two groups, centrally acting and peripherally acting. The centrally acting group, which appears to act on the central nervous system, while only dantrolene has a direct action at the level of the nerve-muscle connection.

Dantrolene (Dantrium) has been used to prevent or treat malignant hyperthermia (severe elevation of your body temperature and muscle contractions during anesthesia) in surgery. When your muscles are tense, blood flow in your muscles can decrease. The decreased blood flow decreases your muscle oxygen level that can cause you to experi-ence pain just as if your heart muscle has decreased oxygen following a heart attack. Decreased oxygen to your heart muscle is the reason you experience angina. Strains, sprains, and other muscle and joint injuries can result in pain, stiffness, and muscle spasms. Muscle relaxants do not heal the injuries, but they do relax muscles and help ease discomfort. Muscle relaxants exert their effects by acting on the central nervous system. In the United States, they are available only with a physician's prescription. Several examples include; carisoprodol (Soma), cyclobenzaprine (Flexeril), and methocarbamol (Robaxin).

Most drugs come only in pill form. However, methocarbamol (Robaxin) is available in both tablet and injectable forms. Muscle relaxants are usually prescribed along with rest, exercise, physical therapy, or other treatments. One muscle relaxant, Zanaflex (tinezanidine) does provide pain relief by decreasing Substance P which is one of your body's pain signal transmitters. This medication is helpful in decreasing pain associated with fibromyalgia. Although the muscle relaxant drugs may provide you with pain relief, they should never be considered a substitute for other forms of treatment like physical therapy. Because muscle relaxants exert their effects on your central nervous system, they may potentate the effects of alcohol and other drugs. They may also add to the effects of anesthetics, including those used for dental procedures. For this reason, anyone who takes these drugs should not drive; operate machinery, or any activity that might be dangerous. People with certain medical conditions or who are taking certain other medicines can have problems if they take muscle relaxants. Diabetics should be aware that metaxalone (Skelaxin) may cause false test results on one type of test that detects sugar in your urine. Patients with epilepsy should be cautioned that taking the muscle relaxant methocarbamol might increase the likelihood of seizures.

Common side effects of muscle relaxants are visual changes, such as double vision or blurred vision; dizziness; lightheadedness; drowsiness; and dry mouth. These problems usually go away as your body adjusts to the drug and do not require medical treatment. Methocarbamol and chlorzoxazone may cause temporary color changes in your urine. Other side effects are stomach cramps, nausea and vomiting, constipation, diarrhea, hiccups, clumsiness or unsteadiness, confusion, nervousness, restlessness, irritability, flushed or red face, headache, heartburn, weakness, trembling, and sleep problems. More serious side effects are not common, but may occur. Anyone who experiences breathing problems, facial swelling, fainting, unusually fast or unusually slow heartbeat, fever, tightness in the chest, rash, itching, hives, burning, stinging, red, or bloodshot eyes, or unusual thoughts or dreams after taking muscle relaxants should seek medical help promptly. Parafon Forte can cause liver pathology (injury) in some individuals. The reaction is rare, but you can develop the following symptoms: fever, rash, loss of appetite, nausea, vomiting, fatigue, pain in the upper right part of the abdomen, dark urine, or yellow skin or eyes.

Muscle relaxants may interact with some other medicines. The effects of a drug may either be lessened or potentiated. When this occurs, the effects of one or both of the drugs may change or the risk of side effects may be greater with either drug. Anyone taking muscle relaxants should let their physician know all other medicines, including over-the-counter or nonprescription medicines that he or she is taking. Some patients for example, receive muscle relaxants from an emergency department. They may not tell their treating physician. If they develop side effects, the primary care physician would not know what is causing any new symptoms. Most muscle relaxants are centrally acting. Central mechanisms of action include activity on the glycine receptors, as seen with the muscle relaxant properties of benzodiazepines, or on the GABA receptors, as seen with benzodiazepines and baclofen. Baclofen has been used to treat the spasticity of multiple sclerosis; it may also be used to treat muscle spasm associated with radiculopathy. This indication is not approved by the Food and Drug Administration (FDA) because the primary activity for this drug has been for myelopathies. Metaxalone has a role, as do other muscle relaxants, such as carisoprodol and methocarbamol. Cyclobenzaprine (Flexeril) has atropine-like side effects. Cyclobenzaprine differs from amitriptyline by two hydrogen ions, and it retains many of the side effects of amitriptyline (e.g., dry mouth, constipation, irregular heartbeats

Some of these muscle relaxant drugs are antispasticity medications used to treat muscle spasms and are usually associated with disorders of your nervous system. A muscle spasm is an involuntary increase in your muscle tone that that occurs when you stretch your muscle. The cause of the spasm is not known but may be related to a decrease in your body's nervous system's ability to be able to control muscle contractions. Drugs that decrease spasms are called antispasmodic drugs and include drugs like Valium (benzodiazepine), baclofen (Lioresal), Zanaflex (tizanidine) or dantrolene. Each of these drugs can exert their effects for a long time. Shorter acting medications will be described below. Botulism toxin administered into your muscle can decrease pain from muscle spasms or muscle dysfunction. These toxins (7 total A-G) prevent release of a chemical called acetylcholine from the nerve ending that goes to your muscle. This action can stop muscle spasms. Botulism toxins A and B are commonly used in a medical practice. These toxins can be used to manage pain associated with whiplash disorders, some headaches, torticollis and low back pain. Botulism toxin can relieve your pain for 3 months. It can take two weeks for the toxin to exert its effects. Botulism toxin injections can cause you to experience mild side effects. These effects may be a fever or mild joint pain.

Benzodiazepines are used for anxiety and seizure treatment, but Valium and Klonopin can both be used for muscle relaxation. These drugs exert their effects by acting in your spinal cord. These drugs are useful if you have a history of a spinal cord injury. These drugs can last for a long time once they have been introduced into your body. Valium should not be used long term. You should know Valium is a depressant and can worsen depression associated with chronic pain.

Baclofen is another powerful drug that works in your spinal cord. This drug is frequently used in patients with spinal cord injury or multiple sclerosis. Baclofen causes less sedation than benzodiazipines. However baclofen can cause some drowsiness. A sedative is a medicine used to treat restlessness. A pump with tubing placed into your spinal cord can administer baclofen continuously throughout your spinal fluid. Dantrolene affects the muscle spasm by direct action on the muscle itself. It is used in spinal cord injuries and for the treatment of spasms associated with cerebral palsy.

Tizanidine (Zanaflex) exerts its effects on your central nervous system. It is frequently used for the treatment of muscle spasms associated with rheumatoid arthritis. This drug also decreases substance P that is a pain neurotransmitter. Because this drug can decrease your blood pressure, you should use it with caution if you have a history of hypertension. The drugs mentioned above can have a long duration. Other drugs are available that have shorter actions. These types of drugs are used for short periods following muscle injuries. These drugs may also be used following surgery. They are not used to treat muscle spasms. Carisoprodol (Soma) has sedative properties as well as muscle relaxant properties. This drug should be used for muscle pain. It will not however, relieve muscle spasms. This drug furthermore, may decrease your ability to fall asleep. Methocarbamol (Robaxin) is a sedative and decreases muscle pain by its sedative action. It has no muscle relaxant effects. Cyclobenzaprine is a drug that is chemically related in structure to amitriptyline (Elavil). This drug does not act on muscles but exerts its effects on your brain. It causes sedation. However, this drug can reduce muscle pain and tenderness. Remember that all muscle relaxant drugs may cause severe sedation. You should not drive a car or operate machinery when taking muscle relaxants.

Baclofen, when administered into your spinal fluid, may cause severe central nervous system (CNS) depression with cardiovascular collapse and respiratory failure. All of the drugs mentioned can have serious side effects. Diazepam (Valium) may be highly addictive. It is a controlled substance under federal law. Valium can be a tranquilizer (a drug that has a calming effect and is used to treat anxiety and emotional tension). Dantrolene has a potential to cause liver damage. The incidence of hepatitis is related to the amount of drug that you have taken, but may occur even with a short period of small doses. Hepatitis has been most frequently observed between the third and twelfth months of therapy. The risk of liver injury appears to be greater in women, in patients over 35 years of age and in patients taking other medications in addition to dantrolene.

If you are taking certain muscle relaxants and experience purple colored urine, you do not have a serious illness.  For example, methocarbamol and chlorzoxazone may cause harmless color changes in your urine such as orange or reddish-purple with chlorzoxazone and purple, brown, or green with methocarbamol. Your urine will return to its normal color when you stop taking the medicine. Because each of these drugs can cause sedation, they should be used with caution with other drugs including alcohol that may also cause drowsiness. Drugs that inhibit the metabolism of Valium in your liver may increase the activity of the diazepam (Valium). These drugs include: cimetidine, oral contraceptives, disulfiram, fluoxetine, isoniazid, ketoconazole, metoprolol, propoxyphene, propranolol, and valproic acid. In females dantrolene may have an interaction with estrogens. The rate of liver damage in women over the age of 35 who were taking estrogens is higher than in other groups.

# 11. NEUROPATHIC PAIN

Anticonvulsant drugs have been used for the management of neuropathic (damaged nerves) pain since the 1960s. These drugs interfere with the total number of pain signals that travel to your brain. In other words fewer pain signals are processed by your brain. The clinical impression is that they are useful for chronic neuropathic (nerve damage) pain, especially when the pain is lancinating or burning. Pain is usually the natural consequence of tissue injury resulting in approximately forty million medical appointments per year. In general, following most injuries, as the healing process commences, the pain and tenderness associated with your injury will resolve. Unfortunately, some individuals experience pain without an obvious injury or suffer pain that persists for months or years after their initial injury. This pain condition is neuropathic in nature and accounts for a large number of patients presenting to pain clinics with chronic pain.

Following any tissue injury (nerve, muscle, bone, etc.) your nervous system sounds an alarm to your brain to make you aware that you have been injured. Rather than your nervous system functioning properly to sound an alarm regarding tissue injury, in neuropathic pain, the peripheral or central nervous systems are malfunctioning and become the cause of the pain. In other words, after your nerve has healed it may still transmit pain signals without any stimulus.. An example is a car alarm. The alarm will sound if your vehicle is being tampered with. This is normal. Now imagine that your alarm sounds when no one is near your car. Somehow there is a short circuit. The same occurs within your nervous system.

Neuropathic pain is a complex, pain state that usually is accompanied by nerve injury. With neuropathic pain, the nerve fibers themselves may be damaged, dysfunctional or injured. These damaged nerve fibers send incorrect signals to other pain centers. The impact of nerve injury includes a change in nerve function both at the site of injury and areas around the injury. Symptoms may include: shooting and burning pain and tingling and numbness. In order to understand the effects of anti-seizure drugs, you need to be aware that these drugs can block the ion (calcium and sodium) channels that are present throughout your nervous system. Ion channels are pore-forming proteins that help to establish and control a small electrical gradient between the inside and outside of your nerve cells. When ions flow in and out of your neuron, this electrical gradient ceases and pain signals subsequently cease to be transmitted to your brain. Calcium and sodium channed anticonvulsant drugs block the pores or channels. When these drugs drop off of these channels, you will experience pain again.

Anti-seizure drugs are frequently used in pain management. It is not known exactly how anticonvulsants work to reduce pain. They may block the flow of pain signals from your brain and spinal cord. Some anticonvulsant drugs may work better than others for certain conditions. Neuropathic pain is a form of chronic pain caused by an injury to or a disease of your peripheral or central nervous system. It does not respond well to traditional pain therapies like opioids or nonsteroidal anti-inflammatory drugs. In neuropathic pain, it has shown that a number of pathophysiological and biochemical changes take place in the nervous system as a result of an insult to a nerve. This property of the nervous system to adapt to external stimuli plays a crucial role in the onset and maintenance of pain symptoms. Carbamazepine (Tegretol), the first anticonvulsant studied in clinical trials, probably alleviates pain by decreasing conductance in sodium channels and inhibits ectopic nerve discharges. Results from clinical trials have been positive in the treatment of trigeminal neuralgia, painful diabetic neuropathy and postherpetic neuralgia with this medication.

Gabapentin (Neurontin) and pregabilin (Lyrica) have the most clearly demonstrated analgesic effects for the treatment of neuropathic pain, specifically for the treatment of painful diabetic neuropathy and postherpetic neuralgia. Based on the positive results of these studies and its favorable adverse effect profile, gabapentin or pregabilin should be considered the first choice of therapy for neuropathic pain. Evidence for the efficacy of phenytoin as an antinociceptive agent is, at best, weak to modest. Lamotrigine (Lamictal) on the other hand has good potential to modulate and control neuropathic pain. There is a potential for phenobarbital, clonazepam, valproic acid, topiramate, pregabalin and tiagabine to have antihyperalgesic and antinociceptive activities based on result in animal models of neuropathic pain, but the efficacy of these drugs in the treatment of human neuropathic pain has not yet been fully determined in clinical trials. The role of anticonvulsant drugs in the treatment of neuropathic pain is evolving and has been clearly demonstrated with gabapentin and carbamazepine. Further advances in our understanding of the mechanisms underlying neuropathic pain syndromes and well-designed clinical trials should further the opportunities to establish the role of anticonvulsants in the treatment of neuropathic pain.

If you have had a direct injury to one of your nerves, you may benefit from an anticonvulsant drug. The clinical impression is that these drugs are useful for the treatment of chronic neuropathic pain, especially when the pain is lancinating or burning. There are seven drugs that are useful in neuropathic (nerve injury) pain; pregabilin (Lyrica), gabapentin (Neurontin), carbamazepine (Tegretol), valproic acid (Depakote), clonazepamm (Klonopin), phenytoin (Dilantin) ,zonisamide (Zonegran)) and lamotrigine (Lamictal). Neurontin is an effective drug for the treatment of neuropathic pain but Lyrica is becoming widely used in the management of many pain syndromes. It has fewer side effects than other anticonvulsant drugs. These drugs can be useful for the treatment of shingles, diabetic neuropathy and fibromyalgia. Reflex Sympathetic Dystrophy, diabetic neuropathy migraine headaches, sciatica, radiculitis, and pain associated with multiple sclerosis may respond to either of these drugs.

If you experience sharp shooting pain, these drugs may be helpful in decreasing your pain. If you experience side effects from either drug, other anticonvulsant medications are available. Oxcarbazepine (Trileptal), lamotrigine (Lamictal), topiramate (Topamax), and zonisamide (Zonegran) may also be effective in reducing pain caused by diabetic neuropathy and postherpetic neuralgia. Lyrica is now FDA approved in 2007 for the treatment of fibromyalgia.

Anticonvulsant drugs are effective in the treatment of chronic neuropathic pain but were not initially thought to be useful in the management of postoperative pain. However, similar to any nerve injury, surgical tissue injury is known to produce neuroplastic changes leading to spinal sensitization and the expression of nerve induced pain. Gabapentin (Neurontin) may decrease post-surgical pain. The pharmacological effects of anticonvulsant drugs, which may be important in the modulation of these postoperative neural changes, include suppression of sodium channel, calcium channel and glutamate receptor activity at peripheral, spinal and supraspinal sites. Because it takes your body time to adjust to one of these medications, your doctor must adhere to the phrase "begin low and proceed slow" which means that you should be prescribed a low dose and this dose may be increased gradually over days to weeks. Anticonvulsant drugs are effective in the treatment of chronic pain but may also be useful for pain management following surgery.

Similar to any nerve injury, surgical tissue injury is known to produce changes leading to spinal cord sensitization which can cause you to have pain after surgery. Gabapentin has been shown to decrease post-surgery pain. Pregabilin is effective for the treatment of diabetic neuropathy and shingles. Pregabilin binds to calcium channels of nerves, which results in a reduction of your pain. Some insurance plans do not pay for Lyrica because it is new and relatively expensive. However, it has been shown to be more cost effective than gabapentin. This drug can cause dizziness, blurred vision, drowsiness, weight gain and swelling of your legs. This medication may decrease your platelet count as well.

Some anticonvulsant medicines can cause a decrease in your platelets which can interfere with your ability to form a blood clot. If your platelets are too low, you will bruise easily. Gabapentin is effective for the management of oral phantom pain following a tooth extraction. Gabapentin binds to nerve calcium channels. The drug is useful in most nerve injury pain disorders. An average dose is 300 mg taken three times a day. Tegretol is a drug that is chemically related to amitriptyline. It prevents repetitive discharges of your nerves. This medication works on sodium channels in your painful nerves. Inhibition of these sodium channels can decrease your pain sensations. An average dose is 200 mg every day. Side effects include dizziness, drowsiness, blurred vision and nausea. This medication can cause various forms of anemia and liver damage. As a result, your doctor will obtain a blood count and liver tests.

Tegretol has been shown to be effective for the treatment of trigeminal neuralgia (facial pain). Depakote is given in a dose of 250 mg twice a day. This medication can cause you to have liver failure. Your doctor will monitor your liver function closely. This medicine is used when the other anti convulsant medications have been tried but failed to provide pain relief. Side effects of this drug include nausea, vomiting loss of appetite and diarrhea. Tremors and sedation may also be associated with this medication. Klonopin may be useful for the treatment of pain associated with the burning mouth syndrome.

Klonipin is useful also for the treatment of lancinating pain associated with the phantom limb syndrome. The drug may also be useful for migraine headache prophylaxis and for the treatment of trigeminal neuralgia (facial pain). The usual dose is 1 mg per day. Side effects include mood disturbances and delirium. Lethargy and sedation may also be seen. This drug has a significant sedative effect. It should be initially only taken at bedtime. Dilantin alters sodium, calcium and potassium channels in your nerves. An average dose is 300 mg three times a day. The number of side effects associated with this drug is significant. Liver damage can occur and the drug can decrease your folic acid level in your bloodstream. A decrease in your folic acid blood level may actually cause your nerves in your arms and legs to have burning sensations.

Zonegran's mechanisms of action suggest that it could be effective in controlling neuropathic pain symptoms. It also decreases sodium channel activity on the sodium channels of your nerves. Side effects can include a decrease in your blood sodium levels, kidney stones, visual difficulties and secondary angle-closure glaucoma. A typical dose of this medication is 300 mg per day. Side effects related to this drug include agitation, anxiety, ataxia, confusion, depression, difficulty concentrating, headache, difficulty sleeping, memory problems, stomach pain as well as liver pathology. This medication may also cause weight loss. A dry mouth and flu like syndrome may also be associated with this drug. Lamictal also exerts its effects on sodium channels. This drug decreases the release of some pain-causing chemical from the ends of your nerves. The reason why you develop chronic pain after having acute nerve injury pain remains unclear. However, it is believed that Lamictal in addition to some of the other drugs mentioned may prevent this transformation. A typical dose will be 200 mg twice a day after starting at a low dose and going to 200 mg slowly. Adverse effects related to this drug include headaches, dizziness, blurred vision and nausea and vomiting. This medication may be of benefit for the treatment of pain associated with Reflex Sympathetic Dystrophy.

# 12. ANTIDEPRESSANT DRUGS

Antidepressant drugs can decrease your pain intensity from an unbearable to a more bearable pain, although they will not completely resolve your pain. Antidepressant drugs are chemicals that go to your nerve connection areas in your brain and spinal cord. Neurons are not physically connected. Signals are transmitted by chemicals that go from one nerve ending to another. These drugs are chemicals that can attenuate the total number of pain signals that go to your brain. As a result you experience less pain. Side effects such as dizziness and sedation caused by high doses of amitriptyline (Elavil) cause doctors to increase doses of antidepressants very gradually over several weeks. Initially only low doses of antidepressants like Elavil are needed. However, the dose needed to control pain may need to increase over time.

Patients need to understand that pain can be decreased by decreasing pain signal intensity input to your central pain processer which is your brain. A computer is an electronic machine that processes information like a computer processor. Taking in information is called input, storing information is known as memory, handling this information is known as processing, and emitting results of the input information is called output. Even the fastest processor needs a buffer to store information while it's being processed. The RAM is to the CPU as a countertop is to a cook: It serves as the place where the information and brain processing tools you're working such as the midbrain with wait until you need to do an activity such as walking, bending etc. to avoid increasing your pain. Both a fast CPU and an ample amount of RAM are necessary for a speedy PC processing.

The analgesic properties of anti-depressant drugs were at one time felt to be related to the alleviation of depression, which can often accompany persistent chronic pain. However, several anti-depressants have been found to reduce pain symptoms in patients not experiencing depression. These agents are now believed to have primary analgesic abilities, which are most likely related to their effects on certain chemicals within your body. Antidepressants decrease the intensity of your electrical pain signals that go to your brain to be processed. Cymbalta is one example. The efficacy of both serotonin and norepinephrine selective anti-depressants would suggest that effects on pain pathways which involve increases of either of these transmitters might contribute to analgesia. Other suggested mechanisms of analgesia involve the antihistamine properties of some agents, increased endorphin secretion, and an increased density of cortical calcium channels. Antidepressant drugs can increase two chemicals in your brain and spinal cord that can decrease the number of pain signals that go to these structures. These chemicals are called serotonin and norepinephrine that were previously mentioned in this paragraph.

A tricyclic antidepressant drug used commonly for pain is amitriptyline (Elavil). This agent can cause constipation and dry mouth, and some patients complain of dizziness when they stand quickly (orthostatic hypotension). Sedation and tremors may also occur. Weight gain and sexual dysfunction have been also been reported. Some people even complain of a craving for chocolate. An overdose of tricyclic antidepressants or related drugs may cause you to experience a dangerous and even fatal abnormality of your heart rhythm. Elavil taken in combination with opioids can cause more constipation than either of the drugs used alone. No antidepressant drug should be stopped abruptly without the advice of a doctor. When stopped suddenly, anxiety, vivid dreams, nausea, vomiting, and dizziness may result. Because of the frequent side effects associated with tricyclic antidepressants. A newer class of antidepressant drugs called selective serotonin reuptake inhibitors (SSRIs) with fewer side effects is starting to take the place of Elavil. You do need to know however, that Elavil may have an effect on acid production in your stomach. Some of these drugs can actually decrease acid production and be of some benefit in patients who suffer from ulcers, reflux, or gastritis.

An antidepressant that is effective for some forms of pain is a combination serotonin and norepinepherine inhibitor called Cymbalta (duloxetine). This drug is effective in decreasing pain associated with diabetes called diabetic neuropathy. Cymbalta however, can make you sleepy and impair your thinking in some situations.

Another class of antidepressants is monoamine oxidase inhibitors (MAOIs). This class of antidepressant drugs is used for significant depression and is not usually used for pain management. MAOI'S drugs have a high incidence of side effects and overdoses can be lethal. These drugs increase the appetite of some patients. This class of drug increases the concentration of epinephrine, norepinephrine, and dopamine in your central nervous system, and when combined with foods such as cheese and wine high in tyramine may cause severe hypertension. For this reason, MAOIs should not be used by people with preexisting hypertension.

Side effects of MAOIs include constipation, nausea, vomiting, dry mouth, drowsiness, and dizziness. Sexual dysfunction may occur. If a MAOI is taken with meperidine (Demerol), a significant and potentially lethal elevation in body temperature can occur. MAOIs can also be associated with liver damage. Blood tests that assess liver function should be monitored routinely when anyone is taking any of these medications. Examples of MAOIs include Marplan and Parnate. The only time that a pain-management doctor usually sees a patient taking these drugs is when another doctor who was treating the patient for severe depression refers a patient.

You should be aware of some of the drugs in the selective serotonin reuptake inhibitors (SSRIs) class. The first drug of this class was fluoxetine (Prozac), introduced in 1987. Overall, this class of drugs causes fewer side effects than the tricyclic antidepressants or the MAOIs. The SSRIs exert their pain modulating and antidepressant effect by increasing serotonin levels in the central nervous system. This neurochemical is extremely valuable in reducing pain. Other SSRIs include paroxetine (Paxil), sertraline (Zoloft), and fluvoxamine (Luvox).

A SSRI, venlafaxine (Effexor), has been studied for its pain-modulating effects in chronic pain situations. This medication been shown to be effective in the control of pain in many painful disorders. The selective serotonin reuptake inhibitor class of drugs can cause nausea and diarrhea. Jitteriness and lack of sleep have also been reported as side effects in a small number of patients. Other individuals complain of sedation after taking this medication. If sedation is a problem, the medication should be taken only in the evening. The drug can be used as a nonaddicting sleep aid. A decreased libido is occasionally associated with this class of drugs. Some reports exist that Prozac may lead a depressed patient to commit suicide. The drug itself does not cause strong suicidal ideations and probably should be hospitalized while antidepressant se suicide tendencies. Severely depressed patients can frequently ha medications were started. An individual who is sincere about committing suicide should be placed immediately under the care of a psychiatrist.

Be aware that SSRIs can decrease the efficacy of the opioid analgesics hydrocodone or oxycodone if taken in combinations with these agents. Both opioids are broken down in the liver to morphine, a chemical reaction that can be slowed by the SSRIs. As a result, less morphine is produced for pain relief.

A relatively new selective serotonin reuptake inhibitor, escitalopram oxalate (Lexapro), is now available to patients that do not affect liver metabolism. This medication does not interfere with the transformation of oxycodone and hydrocodone to morphine. Consequently, its use with these drugs will not decrease the efficacy of the opioid prescribed. This drug should be prescribed if you are taking hydrocodone (Lortab or oxycodone (Percocet). Patients must be told that the selective serotonin reuptake inhibitors can cause generalized muscle pain in a small number of patients. Muscle pain is not associated with tricyclic antidepressant use.

Trazodone (Desyrel) is essentially in its own antidepressant class and is known as an "atypical antidepressant" medicine. Like the other classes of antidepressants, this drug exerts its effect by increasing serotonin in your brain and spinal cord. It is not as potent as the tricyclic antidepressants but it does cause drowsiness and may be used to enhance sleep. Side effects include dizziness and dry mouth. Priapism, a painful, persistent erection, is one of the most serious side effects of this drug in males and may precipitate a visit to an emergency room for treatment. The incidence of priapism associated with this medication in males is 1 in 10,000. The drug should be stopped immediately if there is any change in erectile function.

Studies have demonstrated that antidepressants can lessen the pain of the following syndromes in many patients: phantom pain, acute herpes zoster, post-herpetic neuralgia, cancer pain, cluster headaches, migraine headaches, reflex sympathetic dystrophy, and tension-type headaches. Is one class of antidepressant more effective than another? The drug of choice depends on the incidence of side effects as well as the effectiveness of the drug. This is one reason why your physician may try several different antidepressant drugs to attempt to determine which one works the best for you.

The occurrence of serious adverse effects resulting from antidepressant administration is low. These complications would be rare at the generally lower dosages utilized in the treatment of pain. While cardiac side effects are uncommon, tricyclic antidepressants are contraindicated in those individuals with heart failure or serious cardiac conduction abnormalities. Orthostatic hypotension (decrease in blood pressure following standing) is the most frequent cardiovascular adverse effect, and the elderly are particularly at risk. The sedating effect often observed with anti-depressant use can be beneficial as patients with pain often demonstrate diminished daytime functioning from inadequate sleep.

You may anticipate occasional side effects such as dry mouth, blurred vision, and urinary retention are more likely with amitriptyline use than with other TCAs. These effects are also less likely at the lower dosages used for analgesia. Nortriptyline and desipramine have been found to induce fewer side effects and are less sedating. While antidepressant drugs have been demonstrated as useful adjuncts for the treatment of pain, their analgesic mechanism remains unclear. Initial dosing should be low and then slowly increased to minimize side effects. In other words, start low and go slow with respect to drug dosing. When taken at night, the sedating properties of these agents can be beneficial in those pain patients experiencing difficulty with sleep.

# 13. TOPICAL PAIN RELIEVERS

Pain relievers can be applied directly to your skin. These topical pain relievers are a noninvasive and convenient method for delivering pain-relieving medications. This is especially important and beneficial if you are not able to take medications by mouth. Topical pain relievers include complementary and alternative medications as well as conventional medications. Topical forms of analgesics, or pain relievers, have been used throughout human history. The use of ointments for medicinal purposes is mentioned in the Bible. The purpose of a topical analgesic is to transmit a medication through your skin into your body. The amount of drug that actually gets through your skin is determined by the amount of pressure applied as you rub it over your skin, the area of your skin covered by the drug, the thickness of your skin and the way in which the drug is dissolved, and the use of dressings over your skin. Analgesics are available in ointments, creams, and gels. They also may be placed in patches that may be applied to your skin.

The advantage of topical analgesics is that they can be placed on your skin over the site of your pain. When compared to oral medications, you will have a lower blood level of the drug and will have fewer side effects and fewer drug interactions. There are different types of topical pain relievers. Ointments are semisolid preparations that melt at body temperature and spread easily. Ointments are not routinely used in the practice of pain medicine unless the ointment is specially compounded by a pharmacy. Ointments are defined in three categories based on your skin penetration. One type of ointment does not penetrate beyond the external layer of your skin called the epidermis. Ointments of this class can be used for the treatment of sunburn. A second type of ointment penetrates to the internal layer of your skin called the dermis. The third type of ointment actually goes through your skin to the nerves and ligaments and in some instances into your bloodstream. The latter two types of ointments are frequently used in pain management.

Substances applied on your skin can evaporate. You do not want your analgesic drug evaporating from your skin. Your pharmacist will add substances such as glycerin to the ointment to keep this evaporation from happening. Ointments can be prepared by your pharmacist or purchased over the counter or by prescription. Some ointment preparations will contain absorption enhancers. Absorption enhancers make it easier for the drug to be absorbed through your skin. Azone and DMSO can both enhance the absorption of ointments through your skin. Ointments should be packaged in tubes. Creams are opaque, thick, liquid substances that consist of medications dissolved in a cream base that usually vanishes through the skin. They are less of a liquid consistency than ointments. Gels are a drug-delivery system that usually contain penetration enhancers and are usually used for administering anti-inflammatory medications. The anti-inflammatory medication must be absorbed through your skin to provide you with pain relief. Gels are useful treatment methods if you have arthritic and/or muscle pain. Gels usually are thicker than creams or ointments and are usually clear, unlike creams and ointments.

The concentration of medication in gels is usually no greater than 2 percent. For example, lidocaine, which is a numbing medicine for the control of pain, is dispensed as a 2 percent gel. However, the cream is available in a 5 percent concentration. This is because medications are usually absorbed through the skin better if used in gel form. Gels usually have clarity and sparkle. They maintain their thickness even with an elevated body temperature. Some gels have been developed that may be given nasally. Some drugs are absorbed well through your nose than through your skin. Gels are usually dispensed in tubes or squeeze bottles. Another delivery system for analgesics is a transdermal patch, which contains medication that is transmitted directly through your skin. A patch containing a medication is placed on your skin and remains therefor a specified time so that the drug within the patch can be delivered through your skin to your bloodstream. Local anesthetics such as lidocaine, capsaicin cream, and fentanyl (a potent opioid medication), are some of the medicines that can be delivered through your skin using a transdermal drug delivery system.

Patches should be applied only to areas on your skin that have no blisters or open areas such as a cut. The patches are made of adhesive materials. You should not use the patch if you are allergic to some adhesives. The amount of drug that is absorbed from the patch is directly related to the length of the application of the patch, as well as the area of your skin to which it is applied. The advantage of the patch is that it gives you a continuous flow of analgesic medications. When you take a pill, after it leaves your stomach or intestine and enters into your bloodstream, you receive a high concentration of the drug initially. As the drug is distributed to other tissues in your body, your blood level concentration of the drug decreases. Once your body breaks down the drug, you will no longer have an analgesic effect of that particular drug. However, when using a patch, you will have a continuous release of the drug from the patch into your bloodstream. You will have constant pain relief without the peaks and valleys of the drug concentration in your bloodstream associated with oral medications.

Natural compounds such as herbs or leaves and roots also can be used to treat your pain topically. Aloe Vera can be used to decrease your pain if you have sunburn. The use of this natural topical product for the treatment of various medical conditions was discovered in 1935. This drug is effective for the treatment of skin inflammation as well as minor burns. Capsaicin is a drug that has been extensively studied in both the clinical and laboratory settings. Capsaicin is the active component of chili or red peppers. Capsaicin can be placed on your skin over your joints if you have joint pain (osteoarthritis). The capsaicin first stimulates the small pain-transmitting fibers (C fibers) by depleting these fibers of the neurotransmitter substance called P. After the substance P has been depleted, you will have a block of the pain fibers that cause burning pain sensations.

Observations in Hispanic individuals demonstrates that they did not have mouth or stomach pain after ingesting red peppers. The reason is the depletion of the pain-transmitting chemical (substance P) in the nerve endings in these areas following continual exposure to red peppers. Substance P is also present in your joints throughout your body. For this reason, capsaicin can be an effective pain reliever for the treatment of pain associated with osteoarthritis and rheumatoid arthritis. It may take a week for you to feel the pain-relieving effects of capsaicin. As substance P is being depleted from your nerve endings, you nerve endings still manufacture substance P. As a result, it will take several days to deplete enough of the substance P to provide you with pain relief. Once you discontinue use of this cream, your nerves will replenish substance P and your pain may return.

If you have a neuropathy, (e.g. burning foot pain) related to your diabetes you could have significant pain relief with topical capsaicin. Some pain-medicine physicians have used topical capsaicin to relieve the pain associated with shingles. You may have a brief burning sensation following the use of capsaicin. You should be warned to avoid contact with your eyes and genital areas. It is recommended that you use rubber gloves when applying the capsaicin cream. You should use the capsaicin cream no more than three times a day. Various concentrations of capsaicin exist. Begin with a small concentration that contains 0.025 percent capsaicin. You may eventually increase your capsaicin dose to 0.075 percent capsaicin.

Menthol is an oil that is one component of peppermint oil. This oil in a cream base can significantly decrease your pain. When you place a menthol preparation on your skin, the menthol will feel cold to your nerve endings. While you feel the cold, your pain-stimulating nerves will be depressed. Following the initial cool sensation, you will feel a period of warmth. Menthol products can be used for the treatment of pain associated with arthritis, muscle pain, and tendonitis. Application of a menthol-containing cream may be of benefit to you if you suffer from tension headaches. It can be rubbed around the neck muscles just below the skull. It can be an extremely effective method for the treatment of your headaches. Allergic reactions with menthol have been reported. It is recommended that you test a small amount of menthol on your skin before applying it extensively to assure yourself that you are not allergic it. You should not use the menthol preparation more than three times a day. Do not use a heating pad or a cold pack over the area of your skin where the menthol substance was placed. Some natural herbs and vegetable juices can be used as topical analgesics as well. One example is onion juice. It is reported by some doctors that spreading the juice of a sliced onion over one of your painful areas could reduce your pain. A tincture can be made by putting 100 grams of minced onions in 30 grams of ethanol for a 70 percent solution. There are no hazards or side effects associated with the topical administration of an onion. However, frequent contact with the onion over time could possibly lead to an allergic reaction. The bark of a poplar tree also can be used for relieving your pain. The bark can be used for control of your pain over your joints or nerves or if you have rheumatoid arthritis. You should not use the bark if you are allergic to aspirin.

When externally applied to painful areas of your skin using the poplar bark and leaves, you should use no more than five grams of the drug per day. Either when using these topical natural products, you must follow the directions for the use of these medicines that are contained on the outside of the package or from an insert that may be placed in a box that holds a tube of any of these substances. You should remember that although these are natural products, they could have side effects like any other medication. Another topical medication used to prevent pain is EMLA cream. This cream is dispensed only by prescription. It is used as a numbing agent more than it is used for reducing pain. This is a cream consisting of lidocaine and prilocaine, which are both numbing agents. This local anesthetic combination is packaged in tubes. An EMLA cellulose disc can be applied over your painful area. The purpose of EMLA is to provide pain relief over the painful area of your skin. It is used in children to reduce the pain of starting intravenous lines. Some pain-management doctors advocate its use to decrease the pain associated with reflex sympathetic dystrophy or the pain associated with shingles. This cream should be placed on an intact skin area.

The EMLA should be applied under a bandage for at least 60 minutes to provide relief over the painful area of your skin. This cream is not recommended if you have an allergy to lidocaine or prilocaine. If you have the blood disorder called methemoglobinemia, you should not use this cream. You should not exceed the recommended dose prescribed by your physician. The problem with this cream as opposed to the Lidoderm patches is that it does provide pain relief for your skin but it can also numb your skin. This could be a problem if your skin becomes numb. This means that you have a block of all sensation in the skin treated with this cream. You should avoid causing any trauma to the area, including scratching your skin or rubbing or exposing your skin to extreme hot or cold temperatures until you have complete return of sensation to your skin. It is recommended that you not use this medication if you are taking heart medication. The local anesthetics in this cream can interact with some heart medicines.

Another analgesic cream that is available over the counter is a combination of methyl salicylate and menthol. This is a cream that is effective for the temporary relief of arthritis and pain in your muscles. You should not use this medicine if your skin is sensitive to the oil of wintergreen. You should apply this cream around the sore areas on your body. You should not apply this cream more than three times a day. Do not place this cream over areas of the skin that are broken.

Steroid creams are sometimes used for the treatment of joint pain. Topical steroids are anti-inflammatory agents. Pramoxine hydrochloride is a topical anesthetic agent that sometimes is combined with steroids to attempt to manage pain. This cream provides a temporary relief from pain. You should not use this cream if you are allergic to any of the substances in the cream such as the steroid or the pramoxine. If you develop a rash or blistering, you must stop using the cream. You should not use this cream more than three times a day. Furthermore, do not use this steroid preparation for more than five days. Do not reuse this cream until you have discussed the situation with your doctor.

Nonsteroidal anti-inflammatory agents (NSAIDS) may be compounded into creams by your pharmacist. These creams should not be used more than three times a day. Side effects with the nonsteroidal anti-inflammatory creams are the same as with the NSAIDs taken by mouth. However, the side effects of the topical NSAIDS are less than the oral NSAIDS. The side effects of any NSAID can include stomach upset and allergic reactions. If the dose is high enough, it could affect both your liver and kidneys. These NSAIDs can be very effective for the management of your pain when applied over your skin. The use of a ketoprofen gel and a diclofenac gel, both NSAIDs, were compared at painful sites in a four-week study. The ketoprofen gel gave positive results for the treatment of knee pain and was shown to be better at relieving pain than the diclofenac gel. If you have joint pain, you may want to discuss these facts with your pain-medicine doctor or orthopedic doctor. Aspirin creams also may provide you with some pain relief when applied over your painful joints or muscles. Amitriptyline and ketamine are prescription drugs that may be mixed together to provide pain relief.

Ketamine is a potent analgesic that requires a prescription. Ketamine is a medication that can cause you to hallucinate if the dose is too high. A high dose of Ketamine is similar to LSD in its pharmacological effects. Elavil, an antidepressant can be applied topically to provide you with pain relief. A study in animals has used both of these agents together to treat pain in the laboratory setting. Amitriptyline, which is an antidepressant, has recently been shown to have pain-relieving properties when applied topically. Amitriptyline cream may be advantageous if you do not want to take amitriptyline pills by mouth.

An amitriptyline cream will not help you if you are suffering from significant depression, but can be helpful in decreasing your pain. Some patients complain of being tired while taking amitriptyline. However, amitriptyline can contribute to pain relief in fibromyalgia and the topical application may be a way of avoiding significant side effects that can be associated with oral use. There is ongoing research in this area. You may want to keep informed of the research on both of these drugs through the National Library of Medicine website at www.nlm.nih.gov. The transdermal fentanyl patch system has become popular since it was introduced in the 1980s. This strong opioid medication was used initially for cancer pain management and then for noncancer, chronic pain management. Fentanyl is able penetrate your skin easily. Fentanyl is 75 times more potent than morphine. It produces less histamine release from cells in your bloodstream and causes less itching than morphine. The fentanyl patch is primarily used for chronic or cancer-related pain.

A fentanyl patch can be used for most moderate to severe pain syndromes. In the fentanyl patch, the medication exists as a gel in a drug reservoir. Between this reservoir and your skin is a release membrane that has various-size holes that regulate the amount of fentanyl that is delivered to your skin. The larger the size of the holes will allow more fentanyl to be distributed to your skin and eventually through your skin which gives you a higher dose of the drug. The adhesiveness around the patch keeps it in place. When the fentanyl patch is placed on your skin the fentanyl diffuses through the holes in the release membrane to the surface of your skin. It then goes to the outer layer of your skin and is deposited in a storage area. From the storage area, it is gradually absorbed into your blood-stream. This is the reason that it takes at least an hour before the fentanyl has begun to enter your bloodstream. You will probably not notice any pain-relieving effects from this drug delivery system for about six hours. The patch is usually removed every three days. After the patch is removed, you will still have some drug that remains in the storage area under your skin. If you remove the patch and do not replace it, you will still receive fentanyl for hours after the patch has been removed.

Fentanyl patches come in different concentrations. The concentrations correlate with the area of the skin to which they are applied. The effectiveness of the patch is not affected by placing it on your chest, your back, or your upper arm. An increase in temperature will cause the medication to be rapidly delivered from the patch to your bloodstream. Your skin's thickness also can affect the amount of fentanyl that is absorbed through your skin. The thicker your skin, the slower the rate of delivery of the fentanyl will be. The patch should not be applied over broken skin because the blood level of fentanyl can be significantly raised. There is no barrier to slow the absorption of the fentanyl. The fentanyl patch can cause a decrease in breathing and even death if you receive a significantly high dose of the fentanyl.

Occasionally, you may require medication for breakthrough pain if you do something to aggravate your chronic pain syndrome. For example, if you are using the patch for chronic pain and you go into your garden and do lifting, pushing, or digging, you may cause the onset of temporary pain on top of your chronic pain. At that time, an oral medication can be taken for treatment of your breakthrough pain. Another popular patch that is readily available by prescription from your pain-management doctor is the lidocaine-containing patch called Lidoderm.

The Lidoderm transdermal drug-delivery system exerts a significant amount of its pain-relieving effects by releasing a small amount of lidocaine into your bloodstream. Lidocaine is a local anesthetic. The patch does not cause numbness over your skin but does give you some degree of pain relief below the patch. There also is an effect on the nerves under your skin that are transmitting pain. This patch is used for the treatment of shingles. The Lidoderm patch contains 5 percent lidocaine. The lidocaine essentially does not reach your bloodstream like fentanyl. The lidocaine penetrates your skin just enough to reach the nerve endings that are transmitting your pain. As a result, there are minimal side effects from the use of this patch other than from the adhesive layer of the patch. The amount of the lidocaine that is absorbed from the Lidoderm is related to the length of application over your skin. The patch should be used for 12 hours over your painful area and then removed for 12 hours. If an irritation or a burning sensation occurs around the adhesive aspect of the patch, you should discontinue use of the patch. None of the patches mentioned in this chapter should ever be reused.

You must be aware that the Lidoderm patch does contain methylparaben, which is found in many suntan lotions. Do not use the Lidoderm patch if you have allergies to any suntan lotions that contain this chemical. You should not use the Lidoderm patch if you are using a heart drug to control your heartbeat. Even though the amount of lidocaine that you can absorb is small, it can interfere with some heart medicines. If you are using heart medications, discuss any potential drug interactions with you doctor. If you become lightheaded following application of the patch, you must stop using the patch immediately. Clonidine is another transdermal medication (Catapress). This patch is applied weekly to one area of your skin. The clonidine patch inhibits the release of norepinephrine, which is a pain transmitter. The clonidine patch also is used for the treatment of hypertension. If you have neuropathic (nerve injury) pain or reflex sympathetic dystrophy, the clonidine patch may provide you with significant pain relief. It also can be successfully used if you have pain following shingles.

The application of the clonidine patch can be most useful for pain associated with a nerve injury or inflammation of a nerve. The clonidine patch will not completely relieve your pain if you have reflex sympathetic dystrophy or post-shingles pain, but it can significantly decrease the burning component of your pain. The patch comes in different doses. The usual dose is the 0.1-milligram patch that is applied weekly.

# 14. PHYSICAL THERAPY

Physical therapy is an important modality that can be used to help manage your pain. A therapist will rehabilitate you following an injury. Your strength and range of motion will be evaluated and treated. Your doctor will refer you to a physical therapist if he or she feels that this modality can be of some benefit to you. Physical therapists are highly trained individuals who will obtain a medical history from you and perform an examination on you. Your physical therapist will emphasize flexibility exercises for you and show you how to do them. You have to learn to be able to move your joints without stiffness and pain. Furthermore, your physical therapist will work with you on your endurance and strength. Most importantly, your pain will be addressed. In many instances, a reduction in stiffness in combination with increases in strength and endurance will significantly reduce your pain. Your physical therapist will also tell you how to deal with your ongoing pain and emphasize to you that you should try to minimize drug therapy.

The history that you tell your therapist will give the therapist important information about your pain syndrome, your prognosis, and the appropriate time that you will need to be under the physical therapist's treatments. Your therapist also will assess your behavioral response to your pain associated with your injury if you were injured in an accident or at work. If you have arthritis, your therapist will evaluate your pain input and behavior response to the arthritic pain. For example, your therapist will note if you grimace when you move your joints.

You should inform your therapist about any previous treatments that you have had for the control of your pain, including injection therapies with steroids. Your therapist may additionally want to ask questions about your social history and family history if they may be relevant to your condition. If you have back pain or neck pain, for example, a family history of rheumatoid arthritis is important for the therapist to know. If a family member has this disease, you run the risk of having this disease, which can influence what modality, you need in physical therapy. You should not be reluctant to give your therapist your age. Many conditions occur within certain age ranges.

Osteoarthritis and osteoporosis are known to occur in an older population. Your therapist must know your occupation. If your job involves heavy physical labor, for example, you may be prone to overstress of your back muscles. Tell your therapist when the pain gets worse during the day or notify your therapist if you have increased pain with certain activities. With this information, your therapist can direct an appropriate therapy program for you.

Try to remember where your pain was when you first noticed it and keep a diary of your pain. For example, if your pain was originally in your back and then later it moved to your leg may indicate a disc rupture. If your pain has moved or spread since you first noticed it, be sure to tell your therapist. Tell the therapist what exact movements worsen your pain. Even pain with bowel movements can be an important history fact. A disc rupture can be associated with back pain during the act of defecation. If your pain is worse in the morning and becomes progressively better during the day, this may be an indication that you have arthritis. Your therapist will need to know this information in order to prescribe the proper treatment for you. Providing a good medical history to your therapist will make it much easier for the therapist to prescribe the proper method of treatment for you.

If you have a history of dizziness or fainting, tell your therapist before you begin an exercise program. The color of your skin will be noted by your therapist. Sometimes if you have arthritis, there may be redness about your joints. Your hair pattern in your arms and legs will be evaluated. If you have decreased blood flow, there may be a loss of hair on your skin. Movements of your joints, neck, and lower back will be done to see how flexible you are. Any movements that are painful will be recorded and then will be addressed during your therapy session. Your therapist will decide whether heat or cold could help you with your range of motion or decrease your muscle spasms, which in turn will help decrease your pain. Your physical therapist's examination will emphasize the joints of your body as well as your muscles.

Your therapist will, furthermore, examine you for any loss of sensation in your arms and legs. For example, if you have a loss of sensation in your right shoulder, your therapist will be careful not to apply heat on this area for any significant length of time. If you have limited range of motion about your arm or leg, your therapist will work with you to increase your range of motion. A heating pad could cause a burn on your skin if you are unable to detect the sensation of heat about your shoulder. After your therapist has examined you, the therapist may call your doctor to recommend any further laboratory tests or x-rays. After the history and physical examination has been completed, your physical therapist will determine what is causing your pain problem and will design a treatment program for you based on these findings. You will be treated as a complete individual, and not as just a pain symptom. If your assessment was not done thoroughly, your treatment regimen may not help you with respect to your pain syndrome.

Your therapist may do a muscle and joint stabilization program to increase your strength and flexibility. You, on the other hand, must always feel that you are a main component in your rehabilitation. If your therapist gives you exercises to do at home you follow the instructions on how to do them and do them on the prescribed schedule. Your physical therapist will treat you with exercise and strengthening techniques, but also may complement your therapy with whirlpool baths, paraffin baths, or other methods such as using electrical current. Heat packs can provide you with surface heating, which may reduce the pain in some surface muscles in your back, arms, or legs. Ultrasound is a deep application of heat. This method can relax your deep muscles. Elastic exercise bands and medicine balls may be used to increase your arm and leg strength. The elastic bands can be used to increase your strength, and medicine balls can be used to increase your range of motion and your flexibility as well as your strength. Some physical therapists use traction for the management of your pain.

Electricity can be used to treat your pain syndrome as well. Over the years, many claims have been made for the therapeutic application of electrical current for the treatment of some pain syndromes. Electrical current is applied to your body by placement of electrodes, which are patches with adhesive that stick to your body. The current is directed over the painful areas of your body. Electrical current can vibrate the molecules of your tissues similar to ultrasound therapy. The vibration produced by friction between the molecules of your tissues will increase your tissue temperature. As a result, heat is produced. As electrical current passes through your tissue, some nerves are excited while others are not.

A TENS unit applies electrical current to your body through electrodes that are adhered to your body. A TENS unit has an amplitude knob that lets your control your pain relief. These TENS units are about the size of a pager. The TENS unit patches can be placed over your muscles or nerves for the management of pain both in your muscles as well as the nerves in your arms and legs. You can use a TENS unit for the control of your pain long term without any significant side effects. Some people have allergic reactions to the adhesive in the patches. Iontophoresis is another use of an electrical current to drive medications through your skin. Different medications can be applied through your skin to decrease your pain. Not only is electrical current used for pain relief, it can also speed up your tissue healing. Phonophoresis is another device that uses energy to drive medications into your body.

Traction on your neck or back can increase blood flow to the injured area of your neck or back. However, if the traction does significantly increase your pain, you must immediately notify your physical therapist. Your therapist may instruct you in stretching exercises to be done at home. You must be diligent in doing these exercises provided for you. If certain exercises that you are doing do not provide you with pain relief, ask your physical therapist to recommend some other exercises or range-of-motion methods that you can do at home or at work. Physical therapists can help you decrease your muscle tension. Your therapist also can educate you on how to decrease muscle tension yourself. Most muscle tension is related to the stress of everyday life. While flying on an airplane for example, you may experience stress when the plane bounces around in turbulent weather. You may experience stress in your job if you have to make a presentation in front of a group. The muscles in your body naturally tense up when you are stressed.

Without oxygen, your muscles begin to hurt. Over a long time, you can develop a chronic pain syndrome as a result of your posture. Prolonged slouching over several years can make some of your muscles contract while the opposite muscles can become longer. This could cause chronic muscle pain. For example, if you slouch over a computer you can put pressure on the discs in your neck and back that act as absorbers. Slouching can cause these discs to rupture. You must attempt to balance the muscles in your body. This will decrease your pain associated with increases in your stress levels. When you are standing, sitting, or driving, remember that your head weighs approximately 10 pounds. If you do not keep your head aligned with your body your head will pull muscles, tendons and joints out of alignment. You must therefore, attempt to keep your head in line with your neck as much as possible. Your physical therapist will instruct you in proper posture techniques.

You should also pay attention to your neck position when you are using a telephone. If you band your neck to one side while talking on the telephone, ask your therapist if a headset could be of benefit. If you feel that your neck is stuck or "catches" in a certain position when doing exercises, that cause may be related to a small joint in your neck called a facet joint. The bones in your neck and back stack on top of each other like blocks. Sometimes these joints can get out of position, especially if you slouch over a desk all day. Your physical therapist may be able to help you with this misalignment of your neck.

# 15. CHIROPRACTIC MEDICINE

Chiropractic therapy was established as a profession in 1895. It is now the second-largest primary health-care field in the world. You may be scared of the dangers and side effects of pills and procedures that may lead you to seek out chiropractic therapy. Chiropractic therapy as a profession emphasizes your body's natural health abilities. Many people associate chiropractic therapy with only back and neck pain. However, chiropractic therapy has been shown to be safe for the treatment of headaches, carpal tunnel syndrome, and pain in your arms and legs.

Low back pain may have many causes. In most cases of injury or strain it takes time for your back to heal. Back pain lasts just as long if you go to a chiropractor, if you go to a physical therapist or if you seek no treatment at all. Chiropractic manipulation and conventional medical care are about equally effective for relieving acute low back pain. Chiropractic treatment is based on the concept that restricted movement in the spine may lead to pain and reduced function. Spinal adjustment is just one form of therapy chiropractors use to treat restricted spinal mobility. During an adjustment, chiropractors use their hands to apply a controlled, sudden force to a joint. Chiropractors may also use massage and stretching to relax muscles that are shortened or in spasm. Many use additional treatments as well, such as ultrasound, electrical muscle stimulation and exercises.

Chiropractic medicine can improve your body function and enhance your body's healing powers. Some chiropractors emphasize a healthful lifestyle, a healthful diet, and stress reduction. They will educate you with respect to your lifestyle at each visit. Many times you doctor will refer you to a chiropractor or physical therapist if you have neck and back pain. In many instances your doctor will refer you to a chiropractor, who often works together with a physical therapist working at their clinic. Both of these professions can help you with your chronic pain.The definition of chiropractic therapy is the correction of problems that exist in your spinal column. This enables your body to function at its peak level without medications, surgical procedures, or steroid injections. In 1999, more than 25 million Americans were treated by chiropractors. Not only do chiropractors take care of back injuries, they also can help you with your neck, hip, leg, ankle, foot, arm, and hand pain. Most back and neck pains are the result of mechanical disorders in your spine.

The problem with chiropractic medicine is that it has been maligned for a long time in the United States. However, it is now widely accepted. In Canada, which is under a national health-care system, chiropractic care is included among treatment methods that are reimbursed by the national system. If you have a back injury caused by a twist or turn, you may want to go to a chiropractor. If you have a back injury and need strengthening exercises, your doctor may refer you to a physical therapist. Chiropractic medicine focuses attention on the relationship between the structure of your spine and how it affects your nervous system. If your spine is not in alignment due to slouching or poor posture, this can cause some of your nerves to be compressed by your spine. Your chiropractor will adjust your spine to remove any spinal abnormalities to reduce pressure off of the nerves in your arms and legs.

When your spine is not aligned correctly, it can cause you to experience tension in your muscles that will in turn affect your nervous system (spinal cord and the nerves emerging from your spinal cord). Compression on your spine and the nerves that come off of your spinal cord can cause you significant health problems and pain. In many instances an adjustment of your spine can remedy these problems. Following your initial care, your chiropractor may re-evaluate your progress from time to time. After your spine has been misaligned for any length of time, your body may have a tendency to resume that misalignment again. Therefore, periodic visits with your chiropractor are recommended.

Traction is another method that is frequently used by chiropractors and physical therapists and can be an effective treatment for back pain. Traction involves mechanical forces that separate adjacent body parts away from each other. If you have problems with a disc in your neck or back, traction can separate the bones in your back and increase your blood flow to your injured disc, which can speed up the healing process. If traction worsens of your pain, you should inform your health-care provider so that the traction can be immediately discontinued. Because of the differences in muscle mass between men and women, the amount of traction applied will differ between men and women. If you have a ruptured disc in your neck or back, traction can help heal this painful entity.

Chiropractors treat other entities besides back pain. For example, if you have a carpal tunnel syndrome, chiropractic manipulation can sometimes correct this condition. On occasion, you may not need surgery after chiropractic treatment.

# 16. PSYCHOLOGY AND PAIN

Psychological factors such as your mood, beliefs about your pain and your coping style have been found to play important roles in your adjustment to chronic pain. For example, if your pain persists over time, you may avoid doing regular activities for fear of further injury or increased pain. This can include work, social activities, or hobbies. As you withdraw and become less active, your muscles may become weaker, you may begin to gain or lose weight, and your overall physical conditioning may decline. If your pain persists, you may feel that your pain will never get better. You may then become anxious or depressed. These types of thoughts, along with decreased participation in enjoyable and reinforcing activities, can cause depression and anxiety. The fact that psychological have an impact on your experience of pain does not mean that the pain is in your head or is not real. Most people who report pain are really experiencing it, even if a physical cause cannot be identified.

As you can see, your mind can influence your pain. For example, if you are anxious and depressed you experience of pain becomes worse. On the other hand severe pain can cause anxiety and depression. Chronic pain can impact all areas of your life and is often associated with functional, psychological and social problems. Psychological factors such as mood, beliefs about pain and coping style have been found to play an important role in your adjustment to your chronic pain. For example you may avoid doing regular activities for fear of further injury or increased pain. This can include work, social activities, or hobbies.

Psychological problems can contribute to the belief that one is disabled. As pain persists, you may develop negative beliefs about your pain. These thoughts may make you feel depressed and anxious. The fact that psychological factors can have an impact on your experience of pain does not mean that the pain is not real. Remember that pain is an unpleasant sensory and emotional response to tissue trauma. Your doctor may refer you for a psychological evaluation. You will be required to describe your pain to your psychologist. These tests were described in more detail in a previous chapter. Using descriptive words is one method of describing your pain. A pain-rating index consists of groups of words associated with pain. This index has been incorporated into the McGill pain questionnaire, a type of verbal assessment that uses word descriptors that are valuable in discriminating between different pain syndromes. An example of clinical behavioral medicine is the treatment of chronic pain by "unlearning" it. Some people suffer injuries, resulting in pain and disability, but after they heal physically the pain remains.

A McGill pain questionnaire is a method for assessing pain psychologically. A McGill pain questionnaire gives a multidimensional pain score. You are given 20 word sets that describe a different dimension of your pain. You are asked to select words relevant to your pain from each of these 20 sets. For example, one set includes the words "jumping," "flashing," and "shooting." Another set includes the words "tingling," "itching," "smarting," and "stinging." You circle the word that relates closest to the pain you feel throughout the 20 word sets.

This questionnaire is difficult to administer, takes significant time to complete and can be difficult to interpret. However, it has characteristic response patterns for different pain syndromes such as back pain, arthritis, and cancer. The validity of this questionnaire continues to be studied. The McGill pain questionnaire consists of four different parts. The first part consists of a human figure drawing on which you are instructed to mark the location of your pain. The second part is the pain-rating index that contains 78 words divided into 20 groups. Each set contains up to six words. Five of these groups describe tension or fear. Each word is assigned a value according to its position within a subclass. The third part of this test asks additional questions about prior pain experiences, as well as the location of the pain and current usage of pain medications. The fourth part consists of a present pain intensity index. This aspect of the test requests a pain score from 0 to 5 with word descriptors such as no pain, mild pain, discomforting pain, distressing pain, or horrible and excruciating pain. These words also are assigned different values.

All of the values are added to obtain a total score. All the scores are then evaluated to attempt to assess your total pain experience. The problem with this test is that there is no specific mechanism within the test itself to determine which component truly reflects your pain experience. The value of this test, however, is that it treats pain as a multidimensional experience. There also is a short form of the McGill pain questionnaire that has been developed. This questionnaire contains fewer words and categories than the long form. This test is sensitive to evaluations of reduction in pain experiences. This test is more useful for rapid evaluation of data following procedures or surgery. Your psychologist may administer other tests such as the Beck Depression Inventory test. This test gives the psychologist an indication of any degree of depression that you may be experiencing. These are just two tests out of many. The purpose of these tests is to ascertain how well you are coping with your pain.

One particular psychological treatment approach that has been found to be highly effective in helping patients to reduce pain, disability and distress is Cognitive Behavioral Therapy (CBT). This type of therapy involves modifying negative thoughts related to pain and on increasing your activity level and productive functioning. This approach for pain management has been shown to be highly effective in promoting positive cognitive and behavioral changes in chronic pain patients. Psychological treatment can be delivered individually or in a group setting. Your therapy will be tailored to your individual needs. In addition to decreasing negative thoughts, this therapy attempts to increase your activity level and productive functioning. This approach for pain management has been shown to be highly effective in promoting positive cognitive and behavioral changes in individuals with chronic pain. CBT may incorporate exercise goals set by the physical therapist, or may include recommendations made by the pain management physician for taking pain medications at prescribed time intervals.

Biofeedback is another form of beneficial therapy for pain management done by a psychologist. Biofeedback allows you to gain control over your physical processes. For example if you experience muscle pain, biofeedback can train you to relax these muscles. Biofeedback is a tool that helps sufferers alleviate their own pain. Biofeedback allows you to monitor and fine-tune the connections between your motions and health. . Biofeedback helps you recognize and control your tension and stress. Specifically, it can teach you to release the tension in your muscles and improve your circulation. Biofeedback works by translating subtle physical changes into easy-to-read signals. A session starts when a therapist attaches sensors to your skin that measures the temperature of a finger and/or an electrode that registers the tension in your muscles. The electrodes, for instance, may be hooked up to a pair of headphones that translate tension into sound transmission. When you relax, the sound decreases but when you are tense the sound increases. Your psychologist will help you relax, perhaps by asking you to imagine a quiet, peaceful place or by teaching you a breathing technique. As your mind becomes calm, the temperature in your finger may increase dictates that your circulation is improving. The electrodes voltage can decrease indicating that your muscles are becoming relaxed. You can become aware of your ability to influence your blood flow and relax your muscles. Biofeedback is useful for stress-related pain. Tension type headaches and migraine headaches may respond to this treatment.

In some individuals, hypnosis may help acute and chronic pain. Hypnosis has long been understood to produce varied effects in subjects. Hypnosis may be successful in pain management. Hypnosis has been shown effective in management of pain associated with childbirth, leukemia and headaches. A Viennese physician, Friederich Anton Mesmer, discovered hypnosis in the late 1700's and his technique was called Mesmerism. In England around 1843, the surgeon James Braid revisited the phenomenon of Mesmerism and renamed it hypnosis. His findings renewed interest in the subject, especially in France, where hypnosis gained popularity again as a form of pain reduction during surgery.

In the late 1800's, Bernheim and Liebeault came upon hypnosis as a treatment for physical and functional diseases. Hypnosis can help you control, diminish or redirect your pain to tolerable levels, turn pain off at your will and relax muscles, decrease stress levels and break the stress/pain cycle. In addition, hypnosis may be effective for the management pain associated with childbirth, angioplasty, phantom limb pain, leukemia, headaches and back pain. If you are to have a medical procedure and if you want hypnosis to control your pain, you must discuss this with your physician prior to committing to a hypnotist. Your physician may have a reason why hypnosis should not be used. It should be evident from reading this chapter that a psychologist trained in pain management as well as biofeedback and hypnosis can provide you with a wide variety of ways to manage your pain.

# 17. LOW BACK PAIN

Low back pain has many causes; injury, stress, poor posture, or aging. Many people experience back pain, and there are various treatment methods available. Your back consists of a large number of bones called vertebrae that are separated from one another by cushions called discs. These discs act as shock absorbers between each bone in your spine. The bones stack on top of each other like blocks and form joints called facet joints. The purpose of your spinal skeleton is protects your spinal cord from injury. There are foramina, which are holes in each vertebra. The nerves off of your spinal cord go through these holes and go to your arms, legs, and organs within your body.

Your spine is kept in place by muscles in your back that maintain your posture. Your muscles also make your back stable during movement. You have many muscles in your back. Any one of these muscles can cause you to have lower back pain. In addition to muscles, you have ligaments that attach each bone in your spine to both the one above and the one below. Ligaments also are necessary to give your back stability. Your ligaments contain pain fibers and can be a source of your back pain as well. Most of your lower back pain is usually mechanical in nature. This means that there is usually an abnormal alignment of your bones and/or joints that can cause you to have back pain. Figure 1 demonstrates the anatomy of your lumbar spine. You should note that the discs separate the vertebral bodies. The discs in this model are of a normal size. The nerves come out of foramina and ultimately go down your leg. The foramina are normal in appearance.

When your back degenerates, all or part of your back anatomy changes. These changes may cause you to experience pain. Disc degeneration however, does not mean that you will experience pain. Patients with degenerative disc disease in many instances do not experience pain. Degenerative disc disease is a normal aging process. This process may be accelerated by smoking cigarettes. You should note that the discs separate the vertebral bodies. The discs in the model (Figure 1) are of a normal size. The nerves come out of foramina and ultimately go down your leg. The foramina are normal in appearance.

You have five bones in your lower back that are called lumbar vertebrae. Your spine functions to support you when you are standing, walking, bending, pushing, and pulling. Your back must perform repetitive tasks on a daily basis without failure. Occasionally your spine can falter. At that time, the cause of your pain needs to be diagnosed. Your health-care provider will do a physical examination on you after you give this person a detailed history of the onset of your pain. You will then receive an examination in order to identify the cause of your pain. After this has been done, you will be prescribed the appropriate therapy.

Most of your everyday back pains are not serious. Your back pain is most probably related to a muscle strain or a ligament sprain from doing an activity that you are not used to doing. You should however, never ignore your back pain. You should be concerned if your back pain goes down your legs. If your back pain is associated with weakness of your legs or numbness or difficulty walking, you need to see a doctor.

The rates for surgery in the United States have increased over the past 20 years. The rate of surgery for back pain in the United States is greater than in most other countries. Following the onset of back pain, there can be a recurrence of lower back pain in a person within 1 year and a 75 percent recurrence in a person's lifetime. Sixty-five percent of patients usually recover from an episode of back pain within six weeks. At 12 weeks, 85 percent of those with back pain are essentially pain free. If you have pain for more than 12 weeks, it is unlikely that you will receive significant relief of your back pain. If you have been off of work for more than 26 weeks because of back pain, you will probably not be able to return back to work. If you receive compensation from a workmen's compensation insurance carrier or compensation following a motor vehicle accident, your chances of returning to work are significantly decreased. If you are over 50 years of age, you can expect to have problems with your back and also have limitations in your activity due to back pain. Back pain from heavy physical work is common by age 50. Back pain is an unavoidable part of your life.

If you do a job that requires physical labor, you can expect to have back pain when you are 50 years of age or older. Even people who have not done heavy physical work can begin experiencing increased back pain by age 50. You should realize that it would be difficult to decrease your back pain if you have become inactive. For this reason, you should do aerobic exercise to prevent back pain. You also can use exercise to treat back pain. The muscles in your back must be strong in order to support your back. This is the reason that you must do regular exercise activity. Be aware that your spine can cause you to experience back pain in many ways. You may have suffered minor or major trauma to your back.

Sometimes a disc bulge can press on one of your nerves. A disc bulge is not a disc rupture. However, a disc bulge can press on one of your nerves coming off of your spinal cord and can cause you significant pain. If your pain persists and you develop numbness, you may ultimately have to have surgery to remove a portion of this bulge off of your nerve. In the very center of your disc is a thick liquid. Liquids cannot be compressed. If you bend a certain way or attempt to lift a heavy object in an awkward position, the fluid inside of your disc can burst through the outer ring of your disc. This is called a disc herniation or disc rupture and can cause you to experience significant pain.

The liquid material that bursts outside of your disc is highly acidic. This acidic liquid can cause your nerves, your ligaments and your muscles to become swollen and inflamed and you can develop severe pain. Most of the origins of your back pain discussed are mechanical in nature. However, injuries to your discs between your backbones can cause you to have pain. Remember that your discs are also made up of cartilage as well. It is important for you to understand that a herniated disc does not mean that you will have back pain. In fact 37 % of individuals in the United States have disc herniations but never experience any back pain. A disc herniation furthermore, does not mean that you are disabled or will become disabled. A disc herniation does not mean that you will need surgery. Most disc herniations are treated conservatively with medications, physical therapy, chiropractic therapy or epidural steroid injections. If you do require surgery, you should not expect to be disabled after surgery. In most instances you will be able to return to work unless you have to do extremely heavy lifting. Most professional athletes return back to work following disc surgery.

The surgery rate in the United States has increased over the past 20 years. The rate of surgery for back pain in the United States is greater than in most other countries. If you have pain for more than 12 weeks, it is unlikely that you will receive significant relief of your back pain. If you have been off of work for more than 26 weeks because of back pain, you will probably not be able to return back to work. If you receive compensation from a workmen's compensation insurance carrier or compensation following a motor vehicle accident, your chances of returning to work are significantly decreased. If you are over 50 years of age, you can expect to have problems with your back and also have limitations in your activity due to back pain. Back pain from heavy physical work is common by age 50. Back pain is an unavoidable part of your life.

In some situations, activity does not cause back pain. If you sleep on a soft mattress, you may awaken with significant spine pain. A soft mattress will cause your back to become out of alignment. Chiropractic therapy may be necessary to realign your back which should relieve your back pain. If you develop spinal stenosis (narrowing of the bones of your spine that choke your nerves that run vertical or foraminal stenosis that occurs when the openings for your nerves to your legs become narrow. Activity does not cause this condition, but activity can cause you to experience pain. You have to walk bent over. You will have pain in your calves. Sitting will relieve your pain. This is called neuroclaudication.

When you reach age 50, the liquid center of your discs, called the nucleus pulposus, becomes dry and less elastic. Pressure on your discs can cause them to protrude and cause your discs to keep protruding until they may become compressed around one of the nerves going to your legs. When this happens, it can compress your nerve. If your leg becomes numb and weak, you will probably become a candidate for surgery. You will need consultation with a neurosurgeon or an orthopedic surgeon. Aging also can cause your facet joints to become calcified and the surfaces of your joints can become irregular. Excessive wear and tear over time may make your facet joints become misaligned. If your facet joints become misaligned, one of the joint components can move forward and can again compress one of the nerves going to your legs causing pain and possibly numbness and weakness. A normal spine that has been maintained with exercise, proper posture, and range-of-motion exercises enables you to bend and rotate your back without pain. These exercises will help you maintain adequate range of motion for your back. These movements also can help increase blood flow to your discs.

Cigarette smoking can cause your discs to degenerate. This may be a reason why cigarette smokers have a higher incidence of back pain. Cessation of smoking will not allow your discs to regenerate however. Nicotine can also interfere with the absorption of pain medicines into your blood stream from your stomach and your small intestine. Many smokers who stopped smoking have noticed that their pain medications became more effective. You should also be aware that if you are a smoker and need back surgery, you might not heal properly. Many surgeons will make you stop smoking at least 4 weeks before doing back surgery. When you reach age 50, the liquid center of your discs, called the nucleus pulposus, becomes dry and less elastic. Pressure on your discs can cause them to protrude and cause your discs to keep protruding until they may become compressed around one of the nerves going to your legs. When this happens, it can compress your nerve. If your leg becomes numb and weak, you will probably become a candidate for surgery. You will need consultation with a neurosurgeon or an orthopedic surgeon.

If there is some entrapment of your nerves by pressure from adjacent body structures, your nervous system cannot function properly. If you are overweight and do not exercise and do not use proper posture, your back muscles and discs will become progressively weaker. Your discs can decrease is size. This occurrence is referred to as degenerative disc disease . This is not a disease but normal aging. You will then be prone to a disc rupture if you perform a strenuous activity. This is the reason why you need to maintain a healthful lifestyle that includes exercise. If you still have pain after conservative treatments have been tried, a surgeon may need to do a surgical procedure to get either a muscle or disc off your nerve to relieve your pain. In addition to degenerative changes in the back and joints as being common causes of back pain, the most common cause of back pain is muscle tension in the lower back. Approximately 80 percent of people living in the United States will experience one incident of an aching back at some time in their lives.

You can have chronic pain following back surgery. This is usually a result of how your body heals and is not something caused by your surgeon. Scar can form around your nerves that go from your back to your hips and legs. This is called a failed back syndrome. Repeat surgery is usually ineffective. Slouching in a chair and at a desk also can cause you to have chronic pain by compressing the nerves that come off of your spinal cord and go to your legs. Your lower back has a natural C curve at the lower end of your back. This normal curve is called a lordodic curve. Chronic slouching can straighten this normal C curve in your back. This misalignment will affect your discs, muscles, ligaments, and joints. Look at your posture in your mirror. If your posture is abnormal, you must correct it. If you cannot do it yourself, you may want to visit a chiropractor or physical therapist to help you with this problem.

Be aware that as you age one of the first consequences of aging is unfortunately in your discs. Before your hair turns gray or before you lose hair and develop wrinkles, changes usually occur in one of both of the two lower discs in your back. The lower discs in your lumbar spine essentially do not have a blood supply from arteries to your disc after age 12. The blood supply of your discs must come from the ends of your vertebral bodies. Most of the oxygen and sugar that goes to your discs comes from the ends of your vertebral bodies. Your discs need these nutrients. If you smoke, you decrease these important nutrients to your disc that accelerates the degeneration of your discs.

There are many causes of low back pain. Fortunately, most low back pain can be managed with conservative treatment. Preventive care is extremely important. You should be aware of your posture. You should exercise. If you smoke, you should begin a smoking cessation program. A walking program can strengthen your back. You should have a firm mattress. Alignment of your spine may need to be done on occasion. If your muscles become tight, you should do relaxation exercises. Biofeedback can help relax your back muscles. If you are going to lift a heavy object, you should keep your back straight and bend your knees.

# 18. NECK PAIN

At any given time, neck pain affects 10 percent of the general population in the United States. Neck pain is a frequent reason why patients seek medical attention. Neck pain can range from mild discomfort to severe and throbbing and is experienced by everyone at some point in his or her life. Most of your neck pain is self-limited and does not usually require medical attention. However, if you have serious cervical spine problems such as that seen rheumatoid arthritis, notify your doctor if you have the sudden onset of significant neck pain that does not go away within two or three days.

Neck pain is caused by conditions that compress nerves or irritate the outer part of discs that are cushions between the bones in your neck. Ligaments in the front and in the back of your bones in your neck can cause pain because they have many pain fibers within these ligaments. These ligaments are called the anterior and posterior longitudinal ligaments. The vertebrae in your neck stack on top of each other and are separated by discs. They form joints called facet joints where each vertebra join. The outer capsule of each joint has a rich supply of pain fibers. The outer capsule holds the top and bottom of the facet joint together not unlike a clamshell. If this capsule is pulled or stretched by an injury, the joint can become loose and make the joint unstable. This instability can cause neck pain.

If your neck becomes misaligned, you can also develop significant neck pain. Over time, the bones and joints in your neck can wear out as well. This is called degenerative disc or joint disease or in medical terms is called osteoarthritis. The disc between your bones can rupture. Your facet joints in your neck can deteriorate and cause you to develop chronic neck pain. Your neck muscles can become tense as well and cause you additional neck pain. The bones in your neck are relatively small in comparison to your head. Your neck muscles are necessary to hold your head in a proper position. Your neck muscles must be strong to hold your head up. Try holding a bowling ball vertically for as long as you can. You will notice that your arm muscles get tired easily. The same analogy is true with respect to your neck muscles tiring from holding your head up.

The bones in your neck that are called vertebral bodies contain many pain fibers. If you fracture one of the bones in your neck, you can have severe pain. The tissue wrapper (periosteum) around your neck vertebra can be injured. The fracture of a bone in your neck can cause abnormal stress to the ligaments, muscles, and joints around the fracture as well as injury to your periosteum (an outer wrapper around the vertebral body). Osteoporosis is a weakening of your bones from a loss of your bone density and calcium. This disease can cause small, tiny fractures in the bones of your neck and in turn can be a cause of your pain. Osteoporosis can be a source of severe neck pain. Discs are cushions between the bones in your neck. These discs act as shock absorbers in between your bones. The cushions are important because without them your neck bones would stack on top of each other. Remember the periosteum and the pain fibers contained in the periosteum. Without these cushions, you would have terrible neck pain.

Magnetic resonance imaging (MRI) and computerized tomography scanning (CT) can help your doctor identify any bone or disc abnormalities that may be a source of your neck pain. Be aware, however, that an abnormal imaging study does not necessarily mean that you will have neck pain. It is possible that you can have a ruptured disc in your neck and you may not experience any neck pain.

There is a normal C-shaped curve in your neck. Your neck bones form a C curve with the C part of the curve located in the middle of your neck. The C curve is called a lordosis. The curve is sharper at the lower level of your neck. The curve in your neck determines your posture. If you have a neck injury, the muscles in your neck may pull your neck in a straight line and the curve is obliterated. If you have an X-ray following an injury, your doctor may note that your neck is straight as opposed to being curved. If your neck muscles are in spasm your neck may be straight. Trauma can cause your neck muscles to contract without relaxing which is called a muscle spasm. Muscle spasms compress the arteries that bring oxygen to your neck muscles and nerves. If your blood flow is decreased, acid (lactic acid is formed in your muscle tissue). Tissue oxygen deprivation causes pain. This is similar to heart pain when you have a heart attack. Muscle relaxant medications, massage therapy or injections into your neck muscles can relax your muscles and restore blood flow. This will decrease your pain.

The outer ring of your disc, called the annulus, will contain the nucleus pulposus within its structure. Think of this anatomy as a jelly doughnut. The jelly in the doughnut is held in place by the outer doughnut ring. Be aware that a basic law of physics states that the nucleus pulposus, which is a liquid, cannot be compressed. Therefore, any pressure applied to your disc at any point can cause the nucleus pulposus to spread outward and even rupture through the outer annular ring. When this happens, you suffer what is called a disc herniation or rupture. This pathology may require surgery on occasion.

Whiplash is a relatively common injury that occurs to a patient's neck following a sudden acceleration–deceleration force, most commonly from motor vehicle accidents. Whiplash is the common name for neck sprains. Whiplash associated disorders describe a more severe and chronic condition. It was known for many years that accidents involving rear-end collisions caused more neck pain than side-impact or frontal-impact collisions. This was noted in 1882 with railway accidents. The cervical spine is subjected to a compressive force from weight of the head during a rear-impact collision. The problem occurs when the body starts to move forward and the head remains. Subsequently, the head begins its movement backward and the weight of the head compresses down on the cervical spine.

Most whiplash injuries resolve with conservative treatment. Chiropractic and/or physical therapy are very effective modalities. If these modalities fail, trigger point injections or facet joint injections may be of benefit. A facet rhizotomy may be done if the pain persists. If none of these modalities resolve the pain, a consultation with a surgeon is indicated. When your head is thrown to the side, as frequently happens when you suffer a whiplash injury, the side on which the head is thrown to can compress the facet joints on that side of your neck. On the opposite side the facet joints are opened. Either of these maneuvers can cause you to have a facet joint injury or can cause you to suffer significant pain.

If you have arthritis, osteophytes can irritate or compress one or more of your nerves. Osteophytes are abnormal bone growths. Osteophytes themselves are not painful. However, when they brush over your nerves or ligaments, they can cause you to have neck pain. Osteophytes, if they occur, are usually pointed. If one of your nerves brushes up against one of these osteophytes, or if the osteophytes compress your or irritate one of your nerves which can cause you to experience mild to moderate pain. Steroid injections in and around your nerves can decrease the swelling of the nerve and decrease your pain. Sometimes your doctor may give you steroids by mouth. The problem with oral steroids is that they can cause you to have a significant weight gain. The injection places a tiny amount of steroids at the area of your pain.

The muscles in the base of your skull can compress a nerve that comes off of your spinal cord and travels to the top of your head. This is called the occipital nerve. If a tight muscle compresses this nerve, you can develop a headache called an occipital headache. If you put some heat over the muscle that is compressing this nerve, it can relax the muscle and relieve your headache. Occipital headaches can be treated by a neurologist. Sometimes an injection of a steroid at the occipital nerve can decrease your headache. An epidural steroid injection may also be helpful. Cryoanalgesia (freezing your nerve) may also be of benefit. Botulism toxin (Botox) may also be of benefit as well. Nerves that come off your spinal cord travel to the top of your head. Some of these nerves form the Greater and Lesser Occipital Nerves. If these nerves are compressed from trauma, muscle spasm or degenerative disc disease or facet joint degeneration, you may develop pain that begins in the base of your skull and then travels to the top of your skull.

If you do develop degenerative disc disease in your neck, you will have decreased range of motion about your neck. The decreased range of motion around your neck is an early indication that you are developing degeneration of the discs and joints in your neck. You will have trouble turning your head and attempting to look behind you. Looking up or down also can be difficult as well as painful. Attention to your neck posture and doing daily range-of-motion exercises for your neck can reduce the progression of degenerative disc disease involving your neck. If you have a severe state of contractions of a muscle in your neck, you may have severe pain. This prolonged contraction of a neck muscle is called torticollis. This usually occurs on one side of your neck. Your head is usually twisted to one side with your chin pointing to the opposite side. Torticollis usually results from disease or an injury to your brain or spinal cord. Injuries to the muscles of your neck can also be a cause of torticollis as well. Sometimes an injection of botulism can relieve your pain.

# 19. FIBROMYALGIA

Fibromyalgia is a chronic pain syndrome that affects muscles, tendons, and fascia (a tissue area over your muscle) throughout your body. This disease is also referred to as fibromyositis. It affects about 5 percent of the population, 90 percent of which are women of childbearing age. You and your physician must function together as a team to properly treat this entity. Fibromyalgia causes you to have muscle pain throughout your body, and is associated with joint stiffness and fatigue. You also may experience sleep disturbances and depression if you have fibromyalgia. It can cause many places on your body to become extremely tender. You are only diagnosed with fibromyalgia after other pain-causing conditions have been eliminated as the reason for your pain. Fibromyalgia is a condition that can be painful, but it is benign and will rarely cause you to be totally disabled. Only you can let it become disabling.

The diagnosis of fibromyalgia includes a history of aches, pains, stiffness in 18 or more tender areas above and below your navel and to the right and left of your navel. You may have a history of irritable bowel syndrome and depression as well. You may be de-pressed and suffer from sleep deprivation in addition to muscle pain. You muscle will not feel contracted but will feel soft and tender to light touch. Tender areas can also occur in your arms and legs. You should note from the diagram that these tender points occur above and below your navel and occur in a plane to the right and left of your navel.

If you are like other patients with fibromyalgia, the muscle pain that you experience is probably more common in your neck and lower back. However, it can affect any muscle throughout your body. Your pain can range from sharp or cramping to a burning sensation. Your pain may be worse in one specific area, even though the pain can be felt all over your body. You also will notice that fibromyalgia pain affects tender areas on your body that are symmetrical, or located in the same places on the opposite side of your body. Tenderness and swelling of your hands or feet are also common. Other common areas where you may notice tenderness include the areas under the base of your skull; above the shoulder blade, elbows, the buttocks (gluteal muscle); the front of the neck midway from the chin to the collar bone; the chest; the sides of the body over the hip regions; and the inner aspects of the knees.

It is more common for women to have fibromyalgia than men. Because of this, researchers are trying to find gender-specific causes of fibromyalgia. In general the amount of pain that women can withstand is lower than the amount of pain that men can withstand. Fibromyalgia is seen mostly in women between 20 and 50 years of age. However, it can affect children and elderly people as well. Fibromyalgia may develop after an injury, a motor vehicle accident, infection (viral or bacterial), or after an onset of rheumatoid arthritis. Stressful situations, cold weather and over exertion can worsen your fibromyalgia. As a fibromyalgia sufferer, you may not be getting enough deep sleep. Even in normal people, not getting enough sleep can produce symptoms of fibromyalgia. It is not currently known if a lack of deep sleep is a cause of fibromyalgia. Some doctors think the loss of deep sleep can hasten the onset of fibromyalgia.

Serotonin and norepinepherine are two chemicals in your central nervous system (brain and spinal cord) that decrease pain signals that travel to your brain. Not having enough serotonin in your brain and spinal cord can cause you lose sleep, which can cause symptoms of depression as well as fibromyalgia like pain. Fibromyalgia also affects your levels of norepinephrine, which is another chemical in your central nervous that also modulates the number of pain signals that go to your brain. Another chemical in your body that causes pain is substance P.

Substance P is found in all of the neurons of your central nervous system as well as nerves that go to your muscles and joints. When your muscle tissues have been injured, substance P is released. This event can trigger burning pain sensations throughout your body. High substance P levels have been noted in the spinal fluid of patients with fibromyalgia. Endorphins, substances produced by your body and deposited in the spinal cord to decrease pain transmission to your brain, are known to slow down the pain-causing effects of substance P. The low levels of endorphins in your brain and spinal cord when you have fibromyalgia may be another cause of pain associated with this condition.

It is well known that vigorous exercise can produce endorphins that are then released in your body. Along with decreasing the pain signals that are sent to your brain, endorphins can affect your mood. It is thought that a lower than normal blood level of endorphins may be another cause of fibromyalgia. People with and without fibromyalgia who do physical exercise have noted a decrease in their pain following aerobic exercise. Normal people usually have an increase in endorphins in their bloodstream following exercise. However, you may show no increase in endorphin levels after you exercise. There is increased evidence that fibromyalgia can be genetically inherited. You may even know of a relative who has symptoms similar to yours. The exact gene that causes fibromyalgia has not been isolated, but several genes have been proposed as a possible explanation for the genetic inheritance of fibromyalgia and they are being studied. Research into the causes of fibromyalgia must continue.

It is a good idea for you to keep a daily diary of your activities and pain levels. When you visit your doctor, be sure to take your diary with you so your doctor can see your daily activities such as exercise, sleep, and eating habits. Also be sure to write down any medications you have taken and what their effects were. This will help your doctor determine what areas you need help in the most, and can help the doctor prescribe an effective treatment to relieve your pain symptoms. Let your pain-management doctor know if your primary care doctor diagnosed any new disorder or prescribed any new drug since your last visit with your pain doctor.

It is important that you do exercise or some type of low-impact aerobic activity. Aerobic exercise is extremely helpful in decreasing your pain and improving your sleep pattern. Swimming and water aerobics are excellent ways for you to accomplish this goal. They are some of the best exercise activities for patients with fibromyalgia. These types of nonimpact activities will help strengthen and condition your muscles, unlike high-impact exercise that can actually do more damage to your muscles. A study published in 1996 said that following physical exercise, almost 50 percent of people had a significant decrease in their signs and symptoms of fibromyalgia. Exercise will improve your muscle range of motion.

Most doctors agree that medications, injections, and therapy alone will not be able to eliminate your pain, but rather it will help you to manage your pain and cope with it better. Taking steroids to treat your fibromyalgia will not improve your symptoms of pain. People with other muscle or bone conditions such as rheumatoid arthritis do respond well to steroids. However, nonsteroidal anti-inflammatory medications such as ibuprofen may relieve or at least decrease your muscle pain.

The primary goal in treating your fibromyalgia is to attempt to break the pain cycle. One way of accomplishing this goal is to correct any disturbance in your sleep pattern. Amitriptyline (Elavil) can be an important drug in restoring your sleep. Numerous studies have shown that getting enough sleep can significantly reduce your pain. If you are allergic toamitriptyline, cyclobenzaprine (Flexeril) can be substituted. In some people, nonsteroidal anti-inflammatory medications such as ibuprofen can be successfully used. Amantadine hydrochloride (Symmetrel) also may be used. This medication is an antiviral as well as an anti-Parkinson medication. Serotonin reuptake inhibitors (Paxil) may also have a positive effect on reducing your pain. There are new two drugs approved by the FDA for the treatment of fibromyalgia; Lyrica (an anticonvulsant) and Cymbalta (an antidepressant).

Nerve stimulation is another method of relieving pain that you may find helpful. A TENS unit (Transcutaneous Electrical Nerve Stimulator) is useful in managing fibromyalgia pain in many patients. This small battery-powered instrument has two to four patches that are placed over your painful muscle areas. Electrical impulses will stimulate the nerves around your areas of pain. This stimulation will cause the production of the pain-relieving chemical enkephalin into your spinal cord. Enkephalin will diminish the intensity of your pain signals that ultimately reach your brain. Another useful device that is gaining in popularity is a muscle stimulator. This device has six to eight patches that are placed over your painful muscle areas. The muscle stimulator machine will stimulate and work your muscles until they are fatigued and weakened. It is possible for your muscles that have been weakened by the fibromyalgia to be strengthened this way.

Be aware of the "leaking gut" theory as a cause of fibromyalgia. If large proteins leak into your gastrointestinal circulation, your immune system may become overactive. You can then experience an antibody response that causes you to have generalized body pain. Some individuals that have fibromyalgia from this cause can be treated successfully with a gluten free diet, colostrums supplements or hyperimmune eggs. A psychologist can help you deal with the suffering aspect of your pain. Your psychologist also may want to teach you biofeedback. This is a good way for you to learn relaxing techniques that can significantly reduce your pain. Your psychologist may want you to listen to a CD or cassette tapes at home. Aromatherapy also could be effective for helping you manage your pain. This method is more effective in women because their scent perception is better than a man's. You may also find that hypnosis can decrease your pain intensity as well. You may want to try self-hypnosis as another modality for the management of your chronic pain.

Insomina is common in fibromyalgia. Chronic insomnia alone impacts 10% to 15% of adults. Epidemiologic data indicate that pain, fatigue, and mood disturbance are common correlates of persistent insomnia. Your physician must try to correct your insomnia. A good night's rest increases norepinerpherine and serotonin in your central nervous system. These are two biochemicals that can decrease your pain.

# 20. MYOFASCIAL PAIN

You may have had muscle pain if you were active playing sports or working in your garden. A myofascial pain syndrome is a soft tissue disorder of your muscles that can cause you not only to have pain for a long time, but it can also cause you to on occasion, have some disability. Your overall activities of daily living, including work, recreation and social interaction can be significantly affected. Myofascial pain is pain related to muscle injury or overuse resulting in taut bands and palpable areas of pain that is referred to other muscular areas of your body. The pain can be dull, sharp or burning. You may suffer from sleep deprivation depression and anxiety like fibromyalgia. Your doctor may make a diagnosis of myofascial pain if you cry out or wince and withdraw away from light palpation on an area of your body

Muscle strains and ligament sprains can cause pain in your muscles and can contribute to the onset of a myofascial pain syndrome. The pain intensity of myofascial disorders can vary from painless decreases in range of motion about your arms, legs, neck, and lower back, which are common in older individuals, to pain that is agonizing and incapacitating. This latter type of pain is seen if you are young and are extremely active. Acute myofascial pain can decrease your activities of daily living. If it becomes chronic, it can be a major cause of time lost at work. The good news is that most myofascial pain can be relieved with an appropriate diagnosis and specific treatment.

Myofascial trigger points occur when there is trauma to your muscle or prolonged tension on your muscle from slouching over a desk or slouching over a worktable. This slouching results in disruption of your muscle cells. When your muscle cell becomes disrupted, your cells release calcium. Calcium released inside of your muscle cell stimulates more contractions of your muscle. A prolonged contraction will exceed the available oxygen, glucose, and other nutrients that are needed for the energy to allow your muscle to continue to contract. With a sustained contraction, you run out of oxygen as well as other nutrients. This allows your muscle cell to build up a substance called lactic acid which stimulates muscle pain fibers.

Substances that cause your body to produce pain-causing substances are prostaglandins that sensitize pain fibers or substance P (a pain neurotransmitter) that is involved in pin transmission. These pain transmitters then stimulate nerve endings around your muscle cells. These nerve endings go to other structures in your body. This is why you notice a referred pain pattern when you have a myofascial pain syndrome. You will notice nodular, ropelike bands under your painful muscles when you have myofascial pain syndrome. The lack of oxygen in your muscle tissue will cause some of your muscle cells to die. This will cause scar tissue to form about your muscles. This scar tissue gives you the nodular feeling when you press over these painful areas.

Not all pain in your muscles is from myofascial pain. Sometimes arthritis can cause muscle pain surrounding your joints. Myopathy is a disease of muscles that can occur and cause you to have muscle pain. If you have a disc herniation, you can have referred pain to your muscles as well. Rocky Mountain Spotted- Fever or Lyme disease can also cause you to have muscle pain. A myofascial trigger point in your muscle needs to be distinguished from tender areas around your ligaments as well as around your bone. The diagnosis of your myofascial pain syndrome is made by your health-care provider's history and physical examination and expertise. No laboratory tests are useful for the diagnosis of this syndrome. If you have the myofascial pain syndrome, you will complain of localized muscle pain and tenderness as well as the referred pain. If you have myofascial trigger points around your head and neck, you may complain of headaches as well as problems with your vision. Remember that you can have myofascial trigger points in one muscle or many muscles.

To make a diagnosis of myofascial trigger points, you must have painful areas in a muscle that is noted by your doctor on physical examination. These painful areas must be nodular and must be reproducible. Different amounts of pressure from your examining health-care provider will give you referred pain. If you truly have myofascial pain your doctor will record whether you have a "jump sign" noted on physical examination. This means that when your doctor applies pressure on your trigger point, you jump away from the pressure. Your health-care provider will usually notice a twitch about the area that has pressure applied to it. At the time of your examination, your health care provided will notice that your pain diminishes with stretching or following injection of your muscle with a local anesthetic.

Your trigger points are classified as either active or latent. Active trigger points occur following acute muscle trauma. The latent trigger point on the other hand does not cause you to have pain at rest but can cause you to have restriction of movement about a certain part of your body. Latent trigger points are from a previous muscle injury. A latent trigger point can persist for years after recovery from an injury. Latent trigger points can predispose you to have pain with overuse of your previously injured muscle. Sometimes in cold weather, your muscle will contract and cause you to have pain. Remember, only the active trigger points cause pain. The latent trigger points cause pain when they become active. Normal muscles do not have trigger points that can be felt or have areas that can cause you pain when touched. You should feel your normal muscles. Normal muscles do not have ropelike, nodular areas or tender areas to pressure and exhibit no observable twitch when your health-care provider palpates your muscle. Furthermore, you will not have referred pain with this applied pressure.

You can have different degrees of severity of myofascial pain. Some trigger points are much more sensitive than others. An extremely sensitive trigger point can cause you to have greater referred nerve pain than a less-severe or intense trigger point. Myofascial pain is usually not symmetrical on either side of your body. However, medical conditions that cause muscle pain such as fibromyalgia are symmetrical. Trigger points are usually activated by overuse of muscles. You can stretch your muscle beyond its normal capability, which will cause your muscle to become injured. Bleeding can occur within your muscle following injury, which may cause scar formation in your muscle. Active trigger points can develop in your muscles following excessive, repetitive, or sustained motions. For example, if you work in a warehouse and load heavy boxes all day over months, you can begin to develop active trigger points. Common areas of trigger point pain include your neck, arms, shoulders, face, back and legs.

Emotional stress can also cause trigger points. Stress can cause your muscles to stay in a contracted state. When your muscles are contracted for a length of time as previously stated, you lose oxygen and other nutrients to your muscle tissues. You must attempt to relax and do breathing exercises and range-of-motion exercises to decrease your pain. Heat and cold my help decrease your pain. Myofascial pain can vary in pain severity from hour by hour or from day by day. The stress required to produce pain is variable. Again, if you are under much stress, it does not take much additional muscle stress to produce myofascial pain. The amount of stress that is needed to make your latent trigger become an active trigger point depends on your degree of conditioning of your muscles and your exercise tolerance as well. If you do not exercise and do aerobic activity and are under a lot of stress, you have susceptibility to develop active trigger points.

If your muscle is stiff, avoid placing cold packs on a muscle that may already be contracted. You should use heat instead of the cold. Viral illnesses can cause muscle pain. If you have a virus, do not put cold packs on your muscles. A virus will activate chemicals in your body that activate pain signals. That is why you ache all over your body when you have the flu. Myofascial pain may outlast any precipitating traumatic musculoskeletal event. The pain duration is of myofascial pain is longer in duration than the muscle strain duration. The duration depends on your overall muscular prior to an injury. If you are a professional football player for example, you can have a muscle strain and never develop trigger points. If you are not physically fit, a minor muscle strain can result in myfascial pain. A problem occurs when you are injured, your muscles have developed a way of trying to prevent further pain. In doing so, these other muscles will cause your injured muscle to be protected.

Eventually your active trigger points will become latent. If you rest your muscle and use a splint or an elastic bandage, your active trigger point may revert to become a latent trigger point. Occasionally you may do an activity that will activate your latent trigger point. This not unusual and you should expect this occurrence on occasion. Many of your muscles around your active trigger point can decrease their function, causing your muscles to become weak. If enough of your muscles lose a significant portion of their function, you can develop weakness of an entire extremity. Myofascial pain is caused by pressure over your muscles. When you are lying in bed, you may have some pressure on your body in the area of the trigger points from your mattress. This pressure from your bed can cause you to have pain. On the other hand, be aware that sleep disturbances can cause your muscles to contract and become stiff and can worsen your myofascial pain syndrome. If your health-care provider does not visually notice spasms of your painful muscle, this individual may snap your muscle to see if you truly have a myofascial trigger point. This essentially amounts to pinching and pulling your muscle up. When this happens, usually your muscle will demonstrate a visible muscle twitch demonstrating a myofascial trigger point. This muscle response can also be seen if you have latent trigger points. There are no blood tests that will show abnormalities that can be attributed to a myofascial pain syndrome. X-rays, MRI images, and CAT scans have not demonstrated any changes that can be associated with myofascial trigger points either active or latent. There have been no reported electromyographic (EMG) changes when you have a myofascial pain syndrome.

The highest incidence of the onset of trigger points occurs between ages 31 and 50. When you are over 50, maximum activity could cause you to suffer from myofascial pain. As you continue to age and reduce your activity as a result of pain, your range of motion as a result of latent trigger points will become manifest. Many healthcare providers are aware of myofascial trigger points.

Chiropractors treat myofascial trigger points, as do physical therapists. Acupuncturists, anesthesiologists, dentists, pediatricians, rheumatologists, and specialists in physical medicine and rehabilitation all treat myofascial pain syndrome. The manner in which each of these health-care providers treats myofascial pain will vary from each of the health-care provider specialties. If your pain is not relieved with conservative measures another method that can decrease your pain is a botulism toxin injection into your painful muscles. This drug is a gram-negative bacterium. In small doses it can relax or even paralyze small muscle fibers. The relief from the injection of the Botox can last up to three months. The problem with the Botox injection is that some individuals develop what appears to be fever and generalized joint pain associated with the bacteria that gets into their bloodstream. These side effects should however, subside over several days.

Prevention of myofascial trigger points should be considered. This may be accomplished by doing stretching exercises both before and immediately after engaging in strenuous exercise. This concept may also be used if you are not physically fit and want to work in your garden for example. Do stretching exercises both before and after gardening. This may prevent the onset of myofascial pain.

# 21. HEADACHES

A headache is pain felt within your head, in your forehead, in your temples, or at the base of your skull. Headaches can have many causes. Most headaches are caused by emotional stress or fatigue, but some headaches are a symptom of a disease within the brain. Of the many pains that you can feel throughout your body, pain in the head region is usually the most distressing. Pain in your head can arise in your head itself or can be referred from your neck as well. There are two general classes of headaches, primary and secondary. Primary headaches are those that occur from structures within your brain while secondary headaches can be caused by tumors, infections, etc. Primary headaches have no structural, infectious or other abnormality that could cause your headache. Examples of primary head-aches are migraine headaches and tension-type headaches. Secondary headaches have underlying abnormalities like a tumor, hemorrhage, blood clot, etc.

Some pain receptors exist outside your skull, and other pain receptors exist within your skull. Structures outside of your skull that can cause pain in your head include the skin and scalp over your head, muscles about your head and neck, and the outer wrapper of the bone of your skull called the periosteum. Your sinuses can also cause you to have head pain immediately above your eyes. Within your skull, you have a lining that can become inflamed and irritated and cause pain called the meninges. Your veins can cause pain as well if they become engorged. You must tell your doctor where the location of your pain is. This will help your doctor determine the source of your headache.

Your doctor will complete a detailed history and neurological examination and may order a MRI or CAT scan to determine what type of headache that you have. The purpose of a neurological examination is to exclude any disease or tumor outside of your brain that could be causing your headache. If you have a history of rheumatoid arthritis, make sure that your doctor knows that you have this disorder. Headaches can arise from instability of the first two bones in your neck. Because tight muscles can also cause headaches, your doctor will check the muscles in your neck. Your doctor will then press on the arteries in your temples. If you have tenderness around the arteries in your temples, you may have an inflammation of your temporal arteries. This disease is called temporal arteritis. Your doctor will have you lie flat on the examining table. Your doctor will ask whether you have a change in your headache after your head is lifted. If your headache is originating from your neck, there may be some relief by lifting your head relative to your neck.

Skull X-rays can prove useful for the diagnosis of a skull fracture, cancers, bone destruction, or some shift of the structures of the brain. If you have pain in your neck, your doctor may order x-rays of your neck, with your neck bent forward and then bent backward. This is called a flexion-extension X ray. This test can determine whether you have any instability of the bones in your neck. Blood flow studies may be done to determine whether you have any compromise in the blood flow going to your brain. A decrease in blood flow can cause significant headaches. Sometimes a CT scan is necessary to determine whether you have swelling in your brain or a brain abscess. An electroencephalogram (EEG) study is sometimes ordered to determine whether you have a seizure disorder or a sleep problem. If you have had trauma to your head, your doctor may want a CAT scan, which will show whether you have bleeding within your head. An MRI scan of your brain can be done to see whether you have loss of myelin, which is a substance in your brain. With loss of myelin, you may develop neurological symptoms that include memory loss and difficulty concentrating and have pain in your legs. This disease is called Multiple Sclerosis.

Occasionally a spinal tap is done to help make a diagnosis of what may be causing your headache. This procedure can investigate whether you have an infection such as meningitis. This procedure consists of placing a needle into your spinal fluid. At the time that the spinal tap is done, a pressure monitor can be used to see whether you have increased pressure in your central nervous system. If you have had no previous history of a severe headache, your doctor may need to order tests to see whether or not you have a bleed in your brain from a weakness in one of the arteries (aneurysm) in your brain. A weakness in the blood vessel is called an aneurysm. If you have headaches accompanied by neurological abnormalities during and after your headache, your doctor will want to make sure that you do not have a clot within your brain or a brain tumor. Tumors can cause headaches with neurological abnormalities such as forgetfulness and dizziness. If you have a headache that first begins after age 50, your pain may be coming from degeneration of the discs in your neck. Hormonal changes that can occur with decreased function of your thyroid gland can cause headaches as well. Depression also can cause headaches. If someone has told you that your personality changes when you have a headache, your doctor will want to determine whether you have a tumor or even an infection of your brain.

A common type of headache is the classic migraine headache. By definition a migraine headache is a headache that returns and varies widely in its intensity and frequency of the attacks and the duration. Usually the headaches occur on one side and are associated with nausea, vomiting, and a loss of appetite. Sometimes you may have visual problems associated with this headache. You can have a headache with sensations that forewarn you of an attack of an impending headache. You may have a sensation of flickering lights or blurred vision or weakness in your arms or legs. These sensations are called an aura. Some migraines occur without an aura. If you have migraines with an aura, usually you have visual disturbances. This type of visual disturbance is seen in 90 percent of patients who have migraine headaches with an aura. Migraine headaches can be triggered if you have abnormal response to stress. No one knows what exactly causes migraine headaches. When you have one of these headaches, you may experience mood disturbances as well as pain. You may have nausea and vomiting as well.

Migraine headaches usually begin when you are a teenager. However, some migraine headaches can begin at age 40. Before you suffer a migraine headache, you may have changes in your vision or speech and balance. You may notice zigzag lines in front of your eyes or small specks in one eye. You may notice different lines that come and go in front of your eyes. You may have numbness in your hands. When the headache occurs following these visual disturbances, your headache is usually on one side of your head. If you are seeing lines only in front of your left eye, usually your headache will be on the right side of your brain. Sometimes you can have migraine headaches that occur several times a week followed by a long period of having no headaches. Sometimes your migraine headaches can be incapacitating. Movements such as bending over, coughing or sneezing can worsen your headache. You will want to lie down. Following your headache, it can take approximately 24 hours for you to feel normal again.

If you have a history of migraine headaches, be aware that some stressful situations such as weddings, funerals, or speaking in front of people can trigger a migraine headache. Be aware that there can be a family history of migraine headaches. Seventy percent of people inherit the tendency to have migraine headaches. If you have migraine headaches, you usually have less than two attacks per month. However, 10 percent of patients have attacks every week. Some migraine headaches begin with a visual aura of zigzag lines or a blotting out of your vision or both. Furthermore, numbness of one side of your face and hand, weakness, unsteadiness, or altered consciousness may precede your headache. Most however, are not associated with an aura. The aura can forewarn you of an impending headache. This type of headache is called a migraine headache without an aura. Sometimes these headaches occur on both sides of your head but most occur on just one side of your head.

Before your doctor prescribes medicines for your headache, your doctor must tailor your medications to your type of headache and take into account your disability, your medical history, and your psychological profile. Treatment of your migraines can be divided into acute treatment of the attack as well as treatment to prevent the onset of headaches. Whenever possible, the factors that cause your headaches should be avoided. Stay away from foods that could trigger your migraine head-ache. Cheese, chocolate, red wine, and some Chinese foods that contain the additive MSG are commonly considered migraine headache triggers. If you have an onset of a headache, a mild attack can be treated with aspirin. Nonsteroidal anti-inflammatory drugs can also be used to treat your headache. Ibuprofen is commonly used to treat headaches and can be purchased without a prescription. The new nonsteroidal anti-inflammatory drugs called COX-2 inhibitors (for example, Celebrex) can also be effective for the treatment of headaches. If you have nausea and vomiting associated with your migraine headache, you may need to take a nonsteroidal anti-inflammatory drug by the rectal route.

New drugs called triptans have been developed and can decrease your headache within a significant time after its onset. Sumatriptan was the first triptan drug to be used for the treatment of migraine headaches. Triptans are much better tolerated than the older caffeine-ergotamine medications. Be aware that the triptans are expensive. When you first suspect that you are having a migraine, take your triptan immediately. Sometimes stronger drugs are needed for the treatment of migraine headache symptoms. Codeine and Darvocet are sometimes needed. Stronger drugs such as Percocet have been prescribed for the treatment of migraine headaches. If you have frequent migraine attacks and if these attacks are disabling, your physician may consider prophylactic treatment. Because migraine headaches can be activated by stress, it is important that you tell your doctor what situations trigger your head-aches. Antihypertensive medica-tions such as Nadolol and Verapamil have been used to prevent the onset of migraine headaches. Amitriptyline, an antidepressant, also has been demonstrated to prevent the onset of migraine headache.

Migraine headaches can be hormonally related in females. They are more common in women until age 60 when the incidence is about equal with men. Migraine headaches commonly occur with the onset of menses in women. These headaches may also occur in the first trimester of pregnancy. The headaches can disappear following a complete hysterectomy. After the onset of menopause, your migraine headaches may disappear or at least decrease in intensity and frequency. However, if you receive hormone therapy at the time of menopause, this can prolong your headache symptoms. Sometimes your migraine headaches can worsen when you begin using oral contraceptives. Concern exists about the use of oral contraceptives by those who suffer migraine headaches, because they run a higher risk of stroke.

Another type of headache that you could experience is called a tension-type headache. This also is called a muscle contraction headache even though muscle tightness is not a common cause of this type of headache. If you have chronic tension-type headaches, you may have headaches 15 days a month. For your doctor to make a diagnosis of your tension-type headache, you should have at least 10 previous headache episodes. The headaches could last from 30 minutes to 7 days. You will usually have a headache on both sides of your head. Your headaches should not be aggravated by walking or routine physical activity. If you have a tension-type headache, you should not experience nausea or vomiting. You should not have visual disturbances that are associated with migraine headaches.

Another type of headache that you should be aware of is called a cluster headache. This severely painful headache is not common and occurs mostly in men. Usually the headache is on one side of your head and can be above your eye or in your temple. Usually the headache lasts 15 minutes to 3 hours if untreated. Usually you will have tearing of your eye as well as nasal congestion on the side of your cluster headache. You may have forehead sweating. Your pupil may be extremely small and your upper eyelid may droop. These headaches can be extremely painful. The exact cause of cluster headaches is unknown. A cluster headache occurs more frequently in men than in women. They also occur more frequently in the spring and fall and occur at the same time of the day. There is a 5:1 man-to-woman ratio of cluster headaches. To treat a cluster headache attack, some doctors suggest inhalation of 100 percent oxygen using a face mask. Usually your headache will settle in 15 minutes. If this does not work, an injection of sumatriptan (Imitrex) may decrease your pain. Some studies have even recommended the use of localanesthetics on a cotton swab placed in your nose.

Steroids in high doses can be used to treat cluster headaches. Medrol (a steroid) can be given in various doses and schedules as directed by your treating physician. This drug must be discontinued slowly after treatment for five to seven days. It may take up to three weeks to taper the drug. Nonsteroidal anti-inflammatory drugs may be effective in the treatment of these headaches as well. Sometimes sufferers need to see a neurosurgeon in consultation to see whether there is a surgical procedure that can be done to decrease the frequency of these headaches.

A headache following trauma can be made worse with physical exercise. A post-traumatic headache differs from migraine symptoms in that a chronic post-traumatic headache is usually generalized and permanent. However, it can be made worse by physical or mental strain. Usually this type of headache subsides in 8 to 10 weeks. You can develop a post-traumatic headache with only a minor injury to your head. In fact, the more severe the injury, the less chance you have of developing one of these headaches. Post-traumatic headache is reported more often in women than men. The incidence of a post-traumatic headache can be forty percent following a head injury. If you are over 60 years of age, you could develop a headache related to temporal arteritis. This usually occurs after you have had a fever. You have a burning pain caused by inflammation of your temporal artery on the side of your head. It is usually accompanied by a throbbing headache about your temple. With temporal arteritis you may have a burning pain about your scalp. Jaw movement such as chewing worsens temporal arteritis headaches. This type of headache can be accompanied by loss of vision, which is a medical emergency. The diagnosis sometimes has to be made with a biopsy of the arterial tissue. Steroids are usually the treatment of choice for this pain. Menstrual periods and pregnancies change hormones in the bloodstream, and this change can trigger headaches. Hormone changes in both men and women can increase you incidence of headaches.

A headache that begins at the base of your skull is called occipital neuralgia. The pain from occipital neuralgia shoots up to the top of your head. Local pressure on the back of your head will reproduce your pain. Trauma to the back of your head or an infection can cause pain. Degeneration disc disease may also cause occipital neuralgia. Your doctor may order a CAT scan to try and determine what is causing your pain. Treatment may consist of muscle relaxants, non-steroidal anti-inflammatory drugs, antidepressant drugs, injections with steroids, botulism toxin or local anesthetics. On occasion, freezing the Greater Occipital nerve may relieve your pain. Currently treatment with a peripheral electrical stimulating wire is gaining popularity.

It appears that there is gender specificity with respect to headaches. In men, when their testosterone increases, cluster headaches become frequent. Cluster headaches are can occur at the onset of puberty. In males and females with an increase in progesterone, estrogen, and testosterone, there is an increase in migraine as well as tension head-aches. Be aware that women produce testosterone as well as men. When progesterone, estrogen, and testosterone blood levels increase in your body pain in general increases in both men and women.

# 22. NEUROPATHY

A neuropathy is by definition, pathology (disease or injury) of a nerve or nerves that exist outside of your brain and spinal cord. These nerves are called peripheral nerves. A disease of any of these nerves can cause a weakness in the muscle that it goes to and may possibly cause numbness and pain in the areas to where the nerve travels. If only one nerve is affected it is called a mononeuropathy. A polyneuropathy involves more than one nerve. A momoneuropathy is usually related to a nerve compression while a polyneuropathy is usually caused by a disease like diabetes. With the onset of a neuropathy you will feel a burning or stinging pain in the area of the affected nerve. Sometimes a slight touch of the skin over your diseased nerve can cause incapacitating pain. Your symptoms are usually individualized, which means that your symptoms may differ from other patient's symptoms with the same nerve pathology. For example, if the nerve in your wrist, the median nerve, is com-pressed by tissue, you can develop a carpal tunnel syndrome.

You may have numbness in the area of your wrist, whereas another person may complain of pain or numbness that radiates into his or her finger tips. As a result, the treatment that works best for you may not work for other people with the same neuropathy. Any neuropathy may cause a burning, gnawing pain. You can have some decreased sensation about the painful nerve. Extreme pain from just a light touch can occur in tissues over the nerve. You can have increased sweating, cold sensations, or skin discoloration in the extremity associated with a neuropathy. The onset of your pain following an injury to your nerve can either be of an immediate onset or a delayed gradual onset over weeks to months. Not all neuropathies cause pain. Some neuropathies cause only numbness. Neuropathies are diagnosed by electromyography and nerve conduction tests.

Entrapment neuropathies such as the carpal tunnel syndrome are characterized by abnormal sensations in the area of the nerve as well as pain. For example, a band of tissue at your wrist can compress a nerve going to your hand and fingers that can result in weakness and pain in your hand. You can have a neuropathy that is not painful but it can cause you to have abnormal feelings in the tissue around your injured nerve. This abnormality is called a paresthesia. You have probably heard of a Morton's neuralgia. This can cause a severe entrapment of the small nerves that are around the bones that make up the foot. You may have significant burning pain with this neuropathy. Some drugs can cause neuropathies. For example, the drug Isonizid used for the treatment of tuberculosis can cause a neuropathy. Arsenic can also cause a neuropathy. Diseases can also cause neuropathies as well. You may develop a painful neuropathy related to chronic renal failure (kidney failure). In addition, people who suffer with the HIV or AIDS can have extremely debilitating neuropathies associated with their disease. Cancers may also can cause neuropathy. Your malignancy can cause you to have a progressive sensory neuropathy that usually is not painful. You may develop weakness or numbness in one or several of your nerves.

Carpal tunnel syndrome starts gradually with aching in your wrist that can extend to your forearm. You will develop pins and needles in your hand and fingers. This sensation can occur while you are driving, holding a phone, or reading this book. You may develop weakness in your hands and drop objects. The diagnosis of a carpal tunnel syndrome can be done by arthroscopy, which consists of putting a scope into your carpal tunnel or by a nerve conduction test.. An MRI of your wrist and hand can be done as well. There are no blood tests that can detect a carpal tunnel syndrome. The carpal tunnel is a narrow passage at your wrist about the diameter of your thumb. The purpose of this tunnel is to protect your median nerve as well as the tendons that go to your fingers. The problem is that excessive pressure on this nerve will cause you to have numbness and pain and can lead to hand weakness. Compression of the median nerve in the carpal tunnel is a common compression neuropathy. A carpal tunnel syndrome affects women more than men. The average age of the onset of this ailment is between 40 and 60 years of age. This condition can be caused by any continuous repetitive movement of your hand, such as typing or working with a computer. If you are obese, pregnant, have a decrease in your thyroid function, or have Raynaud's disease or diabetes or renal failure, you are at a higher risk of developing a carpal tunnel syndrome than the population in general.

When your healthcare provider initially sees you, you will be treated with immobilization of your wrist with a splint. This will prevent pressure on your nerve. If this method fails, you will be given an anti-inflammatory drug or an injection of Cortisone into your carpal tunnel to decrease the swelling in your tendons and ligaments within the tunnel. If this method fails, you will be a candidate for surgery. Surgery to release the tissue that is compressing your median nerve has been shown to be effective for the treatment of carpal tunnel syndrome. Another common condition that can cause a neuropathy is diabetes. Diabetes can be associated with a polyneuropathy, which means that many nerves are involved in the disease process. A low thyroid level can also be a cause of a neuropathy. If you develop polyneuropathy, it occurs usually on both sides of your body and usually in both lower extremities from the knees down to your feet. Numbness and abnormal sensations are the most frequent complaints associated with this neuropathy. You can have complaints of burning pain ranging from mild to severe in both legs. On occasion you may have symptoms of pains that are described as sharp, bolting, shock-like pain. Because diabetes can cause you to have a decrease in blood flow to your feet, make sure that you wear proper fitting shoes. Poor fitting shoes can cause ulcers on the bottom of your feet.

Diabetes can cause multiple nerve disorders in your peripheral nerves.. However, some of the nerves coming off of your brain can transmit pain signals to your face and your diabetes can also adversely affect these nerves. This may cause you to have facial pain. Not only can you develop pain in your legs, you can also develop weakness in your legs as a result of your diabetic neuropathy. Some individuals with a diabetic neuropathy can have constant pain. The type of diabetic neuropathy is called diabetic amyotrophy. This entity occurs on one side of your body. It occurs most often in the nerves that go to your muscles.

The nerves that go to your muscles to and from your spinal cord are called motor nerves. The diabetic amyotrophy is a motor neuropathy. The diabetic amyotrophy neuropathy, as well as other diabetic neuropathies, can be seen if you have poor control over your diabetes. Diabetic neuropathies are found in middle-aged as well as elderly patients who suffer with diabetes. Careful attention to control over blood sugar in the long term is the best way to prevent diabetic neuropathy. The treatment of painful diabetic neuropathy has included anticonvulsive medications such as Tegretol. Neurontin has become more popular over the past several years. Lyrica is a drug that is approved for the treatment of a diabetic neuropathy. Tricyclic antidepressant drugs such as Elavil can help to relieve your pain.

An antidepressant drug called Cymbalta is approved for the treatment of diabetic neuropathy. A drug that has been used successfully for thetreatment of a painful diabetic neuropathy is mexiletine. This drug is essentially a medication that is used if you have abnormal heartbeats. This drug has been shown to be effective for the treatment of your diabetic neuropathy. You can anticipate a positive reaction to oral mexiletine if you are given intravenous Lidocaine and have pain relief with this drug. Lidocaine is not only a numbing medicine but it is also a drug used for irregular rhythms of your heart. If you have significant pain relief with the administration of mexiletine administered intravenously the chances are that you will have excellent relief with the oral mexiletine.

Excessive alcohol consumption can cause neuropathies. Approximately 20 percent of chronic alcoholics develop peripheral neuropathy related to their alcohol consumption. The neuropathy affects not only sensation but can affect muscle strength in your legs. When alcohol consumption is discontinued the neuropathy can recover, but the recovery is slow. The alcoholic neuropathy is believed to be due to a deficiency of thiamine as well as other B vitamins. Tegretol or Neurontin or a tricyclic antidepressant such as Elavil can also be used for the treatment of this painful neuropathy.

Nutritional neuropathy from a vitamin deficiency is another form of neuropathy. Nutritional neuropathy is relatively common. Thiamine deficiency can lead to hand, feet, and calf pain. You can have extreme pain just from light touch. You may have some numbness and weakness in your extremities as well. The administration of thiamine can reduce our symptoms. Severe nutritional deficiency can cause you to develop significant pain related to your nutritional neuropathy. If you don't get enough thiamine, you can develop beriberi. This is a result of a deficiency of vitamin B1 (thiamine).

Beriberi is a nutritional neuropathy that is widespread in rice-eating countries. It is noted in individuals who eat polished rice from which the thiamine-rich seed coat is removed. Two types of beriberi exist. One form is called wet beriberi. In this type of beriberi, there is an accumulation of tissue fluid in your body. With dry beriberi, there are signs of starvation. If you starve yourself, you will become too thin and may become sick. Your nervous system can degenerate if you are not obtaining a proper amount of thiamine. Also, nutritional deficiencies in a woman at the time of conception can cause abnormalities in a fetus, which can cause significant harm. Pellagra is a neuropathy caused by a nutritional deficiency. Weakness, tingling, and even pain characterize it. This neuropathy is caused by a niacin deficiency. Niacin is also a B vitamin. Pellagra is a result of a poor diet that does not have enough niacin or doesn't have sufficient tryptophane. Tryptophane is an amino acid from which niacin can be synthesized in your body. Pellagra is more common in corn-eating communities.

Chemicals you may be exposed to can cause a neuropathy as well. Cisplatin is an agent used in chemotherapy to treat tumors. This chemical can cause you to develop a painful peripheral neuropathy as well. The neuropathy associated with this drug can cause severe pain in your extremities. However, this neuropathy is reversible at the end of your chemotherapy. Arsenic is another chemical associated with a painful neuropathy. It can also cause renal failure. Arsenic can be toxic to your heart and can cause your heart to stop. It takes one to two weeks for you to develop a neuropathy associated with arsenic ingestion. You will have burning pain as well as tingling and numbness in your extremities associated with this neuropathy. If you have a severe neuropathy from arsenic poisoning, you may not have a good prognosis on your recovery. Thallium is an insecticide as well as a rodentcide (kills rats and mice). It can also be used to image your heart by your cardiologist when examining you for heart disease. If you suffer from thallium poisoning, you can have pain in your abdomen as well as nausea and vomiting.

There are many causes of neuropathy. An accurate diagnosis in some instances may be hard to achieve. Sometimes, it takes many tests and multiple physicians to make your diagnosis. You should be patient with your doctor if you do not have an immediate diagnosis of your neuropathic pain.

# 23. ARTHRITIS

Most of us will eventually develop osteoarthritis as we experience wear and tear of our joints. Osteoarthritis occurs when your cartilage is worn down and damaged by overuse, sometimes allowing the rigid and brittle bone ends to come into direct contact with each other. Your bones can wear out and develop irregular growths called osteophytes that can interfere with the proper movement of your joint and cause pain. Your joints provide you Arthritis is a degeneration of your joints that causes you to experience joint pain. Arthritis can be caused wear and tear of your joints (osteoarthritis) or from inflammation of your joints (rheumatoid arthritis). Approximately one out of seven people has some form of arthritis, and there are many different types. More than 35 million people in the United States suffer from this disease, and every year the treatment costs the United States billions of dollars.

Inflammation that occurs in your joints can cause you to have pain as well as swelling of your joints. Cartilage is a tough, slippery layer of tissue that covers the surfaces where bones contact each other in joints. In degenerative arthritis, the cartilages in your joints wear out. A joint liner called a synovium lines the inside of your joints. The synovium contains a multitude of pain fibers. When the synovium swells, it causes release of pain signals in the area where the swelling occurs. Approximately 25 percent of people with arthritis are unable to carry out their normal activities of daily living. This means that they have difficulty shopping, driving, and dressing. If you suffer from arthritis, your pain may come and go. More than 50 percent of people with arthritis however, report that they have pain that is constant. If you have osteoarthritis arthritis, you will experience stiffness of your joints in the morning but that the stiffness progressively decreases as you become more active.

With rheumatoid arthritis, your pain will be constant. If you have the rapid onset of joint pain that involves one joint such as the joint in your great toe, this usually signifies gout. If you have a relative who has a history of rheumatoid arthritis, you run the risk of developing this type of arthritis. If you have had weight loss as well as chronic fatigue, you must include this in your pain diary. Weight loss and fatigue can be associated with rheumatoid arthritis. Your doctor may use a needle and syringe to extract fluid from your joints. Your doctor will look at the fluid to see whether it is clear. Normal joint fluid should be clear. If you have osteoarthritis, the fluid can be straw colored. Other types of arthritis that you may have include rheumatoid arthritis or gout. Your fluid may be yellow. Your doctor will examine your fluids for cells. Your doctor also will obtain blood from you. Your blood will be examined for any elevation in your white cells (a sign of inflammation) and a test for rheumatoid arthritis can be done at the same time.

Your doctor may also order x-rays or a CAT scan or MRI of your painful area. Furthermore, it is not unusual for your doctor to eventually order a bone scan if your pain persists in spite of conservative treatment. A bone scan consists of injecting a very small and harmless dose of radioactive dye into your vein. After this has been done, a special camera takes a picture. If you have arthritis, there can be an increased uptake of the radioactive material into your painful joint, showing that the joint is inflamed.

Osteoarthritis is the most common arthritic disease. It also is called degenerative joint disease with range of motion and do support your body as well. To have normal range of motion, you must have cartilage between your bones. This is why you have difficulty moving when your cartilage wears out. Osteoarthritis progresses with age. Osteoarhritis can cause not only pain in your arms and legs, but also in your spine. Osteoarthritis can affect the elastic cartilage in your discs between your bones. These discs between your vertebra in your back act as cushions between each vertebra. You also have joints in the posterior aspect of your vertebra where each joint stacks on top of one another. These joints are called facet joints. These joints can degenerate, which will cause you to become stiff and will decrease your range of motion. Osteoarthritis can occur in your neck, lower back, or n your mid back.

Degenerative arthritis can affect your hips and knees as well. Your knees may become warm as well as swollen. Osteoarthritis also can affect the joints in your hands. You may notice a bony growth about the joints in your fingers. Joint pain associated with osteoarthritis usually begins gradually and progresses slowly over years. Initially, you may have degeneration but not experience pain. With the passage of time, symptoms may begin. You may notice an increase in your pain when it rains or when the weather becomes cold. Your pain may become severe to the point that it keeps you up at night. Osteoarthritis usually occurs in older people. Approximately 85 percent of people over 65 develop osteoarthritis. However, only half of these people experience any symptoms. Obesity puts increased pressure and stress on your joints in your legs. Obesity is an abnormal increase in your body fat resulting in excessive weight. Obesity is measured by your body mass index (BMI). There must be a 20 percent weight gain greater than the ideal for your height and body build. If you are obese, you have an increased chance of developing osteoarthritis. Any excess weight that you carry may cause deterioration of the joints in your hips and knees.

Nonsteroidal anti-inflammatory medications are commonly used to treat osteoarthritis (for example, Celebrex, Mobic, etc.). Steroids injections into your joints can also decrease the inflammation of your knee joints, which will decrease your pain. Your doctor can also inject hyaluronic acid into your joints for pain modification. Glucosamine, which is available without a prescription, has been demonstrated to decrease pain associated with osteoarthritis. If you persist with chronic pain and disability, consultation with an orthopedic surgeon may be indicated to see if you would benefit from a total joint replacement.

Rheumatic arthritis is characterized by redness, warmth, swelling, and painful joints. If you have rheumatoid arthritis, you will have decreased range of motion of some of your joints in your body. You also may complain of stiffness. This disease attacks the synovial linings of your joints as well as the tendons about your joints. If you develop rheumatoid arthritis, you may suffer generalized weakness and weight loss. The exact cause of rheumatoid arthritis is unknown, but approximately 43 million people in the United States suffer from rheumatoid arthritis. Rheumatoid arthritis affects men and women, all races, and all ages. Family history plays an important role in the development of rheumatoid arthritis. Rheumatoid arthritis may result from an abnormality in your immune system. Your antibodies may attack your joints to cause significant degeneration within your joints. It can usually have a slow onset. However, be aware that it can have an acute rapid onset as well.

The onset of rheumatoid arthritis occurs more often in the winter. You probably have rheumatoid arthritis if you have four of the following seven criteria: 1.morning stiffness around your joints, 2.arthritis of three or more joints, 3.arthritis of your hands, 4.arthritis that occurs on both sides of your body, 5.boney nodules over your bony joints, 6.an elevated rheumatoid factor in your bloodstream, 7.X-ray determination of your joints. The treatment of rheumatoid arthritis is to relieve your pain, preserve joint range of motion and decrease your joint inflammation. In addition, your doctor will want to maintain as much range of motion about your joints as possible. Splinting, range of motion exercises and strengthening exercises can be extremely beneficial to you. Occasionally, you may need a brace on one of your extremities.

Usually nonsteroidal anti-inflammatory drugs are prescribed for the management of your arthritic pain. As mentioned with regard to osteoarthritis, the COX-2 inhibitors are safer for your gastrointestinal system than the older nonsteroidal anti-inflammatory drugs. Some doctors prescribe medications such as gold compounds, antimalarials, and sulfasalazine. However, each of these drugs has the potential to cause serious side effects. Steroids also may be necessary to decrease the inflammation of your joints. Steroids typically decrease pain and swelling in your joints and can be very effective. If these methods do not relieve your pain, you may be a candidate for immunosuppressive therapy. Immunosuppressive therapy is the administration of a drug that eliminates or lessens an immune response. Methotrexate is used frequently for the treatment of your rheumatoid arthritis. Methotrexate can cause liver pathology. Surgery is the last resort for the treatment of rheumatoid arthritis and consists of total joint replacement. If your pain becomes intolerable and if you have significant limitations in joint function, surgery can provide you with relief. Joint replacements are now available for hips, knees, shoulders, elbows, and ankles. Disease-modifying antirheumatic drugs (DMARDs) can substantially reduce the inflammation of rheumatoid arthritis. DMARDs can reduce or prevent joint damage, preserve joint structure and function, and enable a person to continue his or her daily activities. Drugs in this class include hydroxychloroquine (Plaquenil), methotrexate (Rheuma-trex), gold salts (Ridaura, Solganal), D-penicillamine (Depen, Cu-primine), sulfasalazine (Azulfidine®), azathioprine (Imuran), leflunomide (Arava), and cyclosporine (Sandimmune, Neoral).Several weeks to months of treatment are often necessary before the effects of DMARDs become evident.

Ankylosing spondylitis is an inflammatory disease that predominantly affects men. Pain usually begins in the back and sacroiliac joint (the joint where the back and hip bones meet) early in life. An x-ray of the spine of a male with ankylosing spondylitis appears as bamboo and is called a bamboo spine. This pattern is also seen on MRI imaging studies. Ankylosing spondylitis usually affects men before the age of 40. If you have ankylosing spondylitis, you may develop arthritis of your spine as well as the large joints in your body. Ankylosing spondylitis is present in 8 percent of Caucasians and 3 percent of African American men. A marker in the bloodstream called HLA-B27 is present in 90 percent of patients who have ankylosing spondylitis. Ankylosing spondylitis has been observed in rats when the HLA-B27 gene is expressed. Usually ankylosing spondylitis will become manifest in a male around age 20. This arthritic disease does occur in women, but the symptoms are more prominent in men. If you do suffer from ankylosing spondylitis, your primary symptoms may be pain in your hip joints. You may have progressive decrease of your back range of motion. You may have some pain in the joints of your arms and legs as well. X-rays have shown arthritis in sacroiliac joints. Over time, your spine will continue to stiffen. The onset of ankylosing spondylitis is gradual. You have a normal curve in your lower back that will become straight. You may have difficulty expanding your chest to take a breath.

If your ankylosing spondylitis worsens, your entire spine may become fused, which restricts your motion about your spine in all directions. The earliest x-ray changes usually occur in your sacroiliac joints. Erosion of these joints becomes evident. The outer rings of your discs in your spine become calcified. Furthermore, calcification of the vertical ligaments that run in front and back of your vertebral bones occurs. When this happens, if you have an x-ray of your spine, it will appear as a bamboo stick. Remember that rheumatoid arthritis affects mostly small joints. Ankylosing spondylitis affects large joints. Osteoarthritis does not usually affect your sacroiliac joints. If you have ankylosing spondylitis, physical therapy and nonsteroidal anti-inflammatory drugs are important for the treatment of the pain associated with this disease. No treatment is currently available that will eradicate ankylosing spondylitis. Occasionally stronger analgesics such as opioids are needed to control your pain. Sulfasalazine is sometimes useful for pain for arthritis in your arms and legs. The problem with ankylosing spondylitis is that you can have pain that is severe over decades of your life. The severity of the pain associated with this disease varies greatly. Approximately 10 percent of patients have disability so severe that they are unable to return to work after 10 years.

Gout is one of the most painful arthritic diseases. Gout results from the formation crystals of uric acid that are deposited into joint spaces between your bones. These uric acid crystals deposited into your joints cause inflammation with swelling, redness, and warmth about your joint. Gouty arthritis comprises 5 percent of all cases of arthritis. We all have the formation of uric acid in our bodies. Uric acid is formed in your body from the breakdown of chemicals called purines that are found in many foods. You should avoid foods that will elevate your uric acid blood level. If you have a history of gout, avoid excessive meat and seafood in your diet. Do not eat gravies. Avoid yeast products, including beer and other alcoholic beverages. You must also avoid oatmeal, asparagus, cauliflower, and mushrooms.

Uric acid is dissolved in your bloodstream and is excreted through the kidneys. If your kidneys do not eliminate enough uric acid from your bloodstream, the uric acid will increase in your bloodstream. If you eat a lot of liver, beans, or peas, you may increase the uric acid in your bloodstream. If the uric acid forms crystals and deposits these crystals into your joints, gout will develop. In many people, the uric acid deposits affect the joints in their great toes. The big toe is affected in approximately 75 percent of people suffering gout. The ankles, heels, knees, wrists, and fingers may also be affected by gouty arthritis.

If you have a family history of gouty arthritis, you run the risk of developing this disease. Gout is more common in men than in women and is more common in adults than in children. Obesity increases the risk of developing gout. An excess consumption of alcohol also interferes with the excretion of uric acid from your body. The increased uric acid that occurs from excessive alcohol consumption can form crystals and deposit these crystals into your joints. Adult men between the ages of 40 and 50 are most likely to develop gout. Gout is occasionally seen in women. It rarely occurs before menopause. For some reason, people who have had organ transplants are more susceptible to gout. A diagnosis of gout can be made by withdrawing fluid from your painful joints and analyzing the fluid for uric acid. When your gout attack is severe, you may be totally incapacitated. If your gout is not treated, you may develop severe pathology of your affected joints. The prevalence of gout for men is approximately 14 cases per 1,000 men, whereas the prevalence in women is approximately 6 cases per 1,000 women. Estrogen hormones noted in women can help the body eliminate uric acid. For this reason, gout is rarely seen in premenopausal women.

When a gout attack occurs, the maximum pain associated with the gout usually occurs in approximately the first 10 hours. In general, attacks resolve in less than 14 days. Uric acid crystals can not only be deposited in your joints, they can also form in your soft tissues. A collection of uric acid crystals in your tissues can form a lump (called a tophi), often noted on the outer edges of your forearms. Be aware that if you have gout, you have an increased risk of developing kidney stones. These stones are usually composed of uric acid. If you have gout, you also have a higher risk of developing a kidney disease. Finding uric acid crystals in the fluid of your joints makes the diagnosis of gout. Uric acid crystals are usually formed when your uric acid level exceeds 6.8 mg/dL.

Sometimes overproduction of uric acid is related to a genetic disorder. Excessive exercise can also increase uric acid, as can obesity. Starvation or dehydration can increase uric acid, too. Thyroid disease can also increase uric acid. Diuretics (medications that make you urinate, such as furosemide [Lasix] and hydrochlorthiazide [or HCTZ], a common blood pressure medicine) and cyclosporine A (an immunosuppressive medicine) can increase the uric acid concentration in the bloodstream. The initial treatment of gout may include nonsteroidal anti-inflammatory medications or steroids or colchicine. The use of COX-2 inhibitors is under investigation. Steroids can be used to treat gout and can be given orally or by injection into your muscle.

# 24. OSTEOPOROSIS

If you suffer from osteoporosis, you will have a progressive reduction in the density of your bones. The normal composition of your bones is preserved. Osteoporosis affects 20 million Americans and results in more than 1.3 million bone fractures in the United States every year. In a lifetime, women lose more than half of their spongy bone, which comprises the center of bones, and approximately 30 percent of the nonspongy (compact) bone, which composes the outer aspect of these bones. Approximately 30 percent of all postmenopausal Caucasian women will suffer from fractures related to osteoporosis. More than one third of all women and one sixth of all men over 65 years of age will sustain a hip fracture. During your lifetime, bone is constantly being made and is constantly being lost. In normal circumstances, the production and reduction of your bone is balanced. Osteoporosis can result if you do not make enough bone or if you have an accelerated decrease in your bone minerals and the matrix structure (the components of your bone which make your bones hard) of your bone or both.

Genetics can affect differences in bone density and these differences are the result of a gene that is linked to your vitamin D receptor gene. Variations of the vitamin D receptor gene result in differences in bone density changes of 10 percent to 12 percent in osteoporosis-prone individuals. Your bone density will continue to increase throughout your life until you reach an age where your bone density becomes stable. When you approach 40, your bone density can begin to decline. Bone density decreases are noted in women before menopause. In men, a decrease in their bone density occurs somewhere between 20 to 40 years of age. In women, after menopause has occurred, the rate of bone loss accelerates.

Osteoporosis is usually diagnosed when a fracture occurs. Fractures may occur in your vertebra (compression fracture). However, your wrists, hips, ribs, pelvic bone, and your leg bones can sustain fractures. The bones in your spine can have a loss of height, which is called a compression fracture. If you have osteoporosis, your bones become more porous. This means that the bones in your body develop holes, which in turn weaken the structure of your bones. All of your bones can be affected, and each of your bones can be at an increased risk for a fracture. If you have a low calcium intake and are not physically active, you are also at risk of developing osteoporosis.

Hyperthyroidism and hyperparathyroidism in addition to excessive cortisone (a steroid) may be causes of osteoporosis. It is important for your body to absorb calcium through your gastrointestinal system. If you have a history of a gastrectomy (removal of a portion of your stomach), cirrhosis of the liver, or any other gastrointestinal malabsorption syndrome, you are more prone to develop osteoporosis. If you have a history of multiple myeloma or leukemia, you may develop osteoporosis. The exact cause of this finding is presently unknown. Alcohol can contribute to your development of osteoporosis. Chemotherapy can also cause osteoporosis. Steroid use has been implicated as a cause of osteoporosis as well. A plain X-ray cannot make a diagnosis of osteoporosis. You will need a DEXA for a true diagnosis.

Osteoporosis can cause your vertebra to compress. This is called a compression fracture. Essentially your vertebra collapses. This disease can be very painful. If you have a vertebral compression in your mid back, for example, there will usually be a decrease in the height of your affected (compressed) bone that can be seen on X-ray. Sometimes a bone scan is needed to diagnosis osteoporosis. If you have a bone scan, a doctor will inject a radioactive material into your vein. You will have a picture of your body taken by a special camera. Compression fractures, which were not diagnosed by other means, can be detected by a bone scan.

Osteoporosis can also be diagnosed by measuring your bone mineral density. Your bone density value will be compared to a normal value that is noted for young adults of your same sex. A bone density test can predict the probability of you developing a fracture related to your bone density value. Quantitative computed tomography can also be used and is effective for diagnosing osteoporosis because it will not only measure your bone mineral density, but this test can also measure the density of your spongy bone within your back and hip bones. However, this test is expensive and will expose you to radiation. Different types of tests are being used and being developed to diagnosis osteoporosis. Bone scanning can be useful for the diagnosis of compression fractures. If you have a decreased bone density, your doctor should attempt to determine the cause of your osteoporosis.

Sometimes your doctor needs to obtain blood samples from you for further testing. Your doctor may take some blood from you to be sent to a lab to measure the calcium, organic phosphate, and alkaline phosphatase in your bloodstream. These minerals are usually normal if you have osteoporosis. However, your alkaline phosphate may be higher if you have a fracture. Vitamin D can help you increase your calcium absorption through your gastrointestinal tract by up to 65 percent.

Smoking on the other hand, increases the rate of bone loss. Hip and spinal bone fractures are higher in men and women who smoke. Nicotine can inhibit absorption of calcium that is needed for bone health. Osteoporosis in men can be diagnosis by a bone mass measurement. This is a special type of x-ray that emits a trace amount of radiation. Middle-aged men who have complaints of back or hip pain may be candidates for a bone mass measurement as well as a measurement of the testosterone in their bloodstream. As previously stated, absorption of calcium from your gastrointestinal system decreases with age. The United Stated recommended dietary allowance of calcium is up to 1,000 milligrams per day. Calcium can retard your osteoporosis but cannot completely stop it. An increase in calcium in your bloodstream may not protect you from compression fractures of the bones in your spine. Calcium therapy can help you if you are a woman and postmenopausal. Some endocrinologists have recommended that if you are postmenopausal that you should consume 1,500 milligrams per day of calcium.

Calcitonin is another drug that you could possibly take to prevent bone loss in your vertebral bodies throughout your spine. Calcitonin is most effective in early and late menopause. Calcitonin is available for intranasal use. Calcitonin has been shown to produce pain-relieving effects. Calcitonin is most useful if you have a history of osteoporosis and have chronic pain related to fractures related to your osteoporosis. If you have had a fracture of one of the bones in your spine, treatment that puts bone cement into your bone can be used to treat any compression fracture that you may have. The techniques that use this cement are called vertebroplasty and kyphoplasty. Vertebroplasty involves the injection of bone cement into your vertebral bones. Kyphyplasty introduces a surgical instrument into one of the bones in your spine with intent to elevate the compressed bone.

When this instrument is withdrawn, the space left is filled with bone cement. Each of these procedures remains to be studied.

Bisphosphonates are an important class of drug for the treatment of osteoporosis. These drugs can increase the minerals in the bones throughout your body. Furthermore, the chance of you having a vertebral fracture is decreased if you are in late menopause. Examples of these drugs include etidronate and alendronate. Further research is being done with respect to these drugs in the prevention of bone fractures. However, these drugs will not reverse osteoporosis. There are other drugs available for women who have osteoporosis. Fosamax and Actonel are two of the drugs commonly used to decrease the progression of osteoporosis. Fosamax slows the cycle of bone breakdown. If the rate of bone breakdown is decreased, there is a reduced chance of you having a fracture.

# 25. SHINGLES

Shingles is a painful disease that is caused by the same virus (herpes zoster virus) that caused chickenpox when you were a child. This virus is rendered dormant by your immune system when your body has healed from the chicken pox infection. This same virus may affect some of the nerves that go out of your spinal cord to your chest or face. One or more nerves can be affected. Shingles occurs in those patients who have had chickenpox. Usually the shingles pain stays on one side of your body. The shingles virus will remain in a nerve after your chickenpox has healed. This area is called your dorsal root ganglia. Refer to chapter 2. (Pain Overview). This virus is dormant but typically reactivates when you age. This reactivation usually occurs after your immune system has been weakened, usually by another viral infection such as the flu or common cold. If you have cancer, you may be prone to develop shingles as well.

Sometimes there is no known reason why you develop shingles. If you have had contact with an individual who has active chicken pox, there is a chance that you could develop shingles. However, this scenario is rare. You need to be aware that shingles does not increase during seasonal chicken pox outbreaks. When the virus is reactivated in your dorsal root ganglia, it goes along your nerves to your nerve endings. The virus at this time will cause your skin to develop painful skin lesions. You need to be aware that this virus can affect any part of your central nervous system. In rare cases, this virus can even affect your brain; this is called encephalitis. The virus has been reported in some cases to affect the sympathetic ganglia as well, which can cause severe burning pain. This will cause you to have symptoms that mimic reflex sympathetic dystrophy.

Following a chicken pox infection, antibodies are made in your body to fight the chicken pox virus. This is the reason why you usually do not get chicken pox again. However, if your immune system is compromised for any reason, your body's ability to combat the virus is greatly reduced. This is the reason why you may develop shingles. If your immune system appears to be attacked, your body will immediately fight the shingles virus by producing antibodies to the virus. After you have had the onset of shingles, you may develop post-herpetic neuralgia. This is a chronic pain syndrome that occurs following the onset of shingles. When you have the onset of shingles, you will have blisters as well as burning sensations in your skin where the infected nerves run. When you develop post-herpetic neuralgia, which can persist for years, after your skin lesions have healed.

If you are between the ages of 40 and 60, the chances of you developing post-herpetic neuralgia are 20 percent. If you are over 60 years of age, your chance of developing post-herpetic neuralgia will increase to 50 percent. Post-herpetic neuralgia is a difficult entity to treat. Post-herpetic neuralgia can cause you to have agonizing pain as well as suffering. Some individuals have even committed suicide to escape this terrible pain. Sometimes you can develop burning pain associated with the herpes zoster virus. However, it may be some time before your skin lesions appear. Before you develop a skin rash, the diagnosis of herpes zoster is difficult to make. After your skin lesions erupt, the diagnosis is easier to make. If you have pain in your mid chest, you may be incorrectly diagnosed with a coronary artery disease or pneumonia. If your doctor wants to confirm your diagnosis, the virus should be isolated from your pustules no later than seven days after they erupted. Be aware that if you have severe burning pain that develops on one side of your body, you may or may not have a skin eruption but you can have shingles. Sometimes the lack of a skin eruption confuses doctors as to whether you actually have the onset of shingles, because skin lesions are so common. If you do develop skin eruptions, the lesions will begin as redness. The redness over your skin will turn to blisters. The blisters can form pus. Eventually these lesions on your skin break down. A crust then forms. If the virus affects your skin, in addition to your nerves, you may develop scars as well as loss of skin pigment about the infected site.

Also be aware that the virus can travel to your eyes. If you or anyone in your family has developed shingles and begins to complain of eye pain, this is a medical emergency. You must contact an ophthalmologist immediately. If left untreated, the virus may blind you. Shingles may be preceded by other events. Be aware that psychological stress can also trigger the onset of shingles. If you have a history of a prolonged use of steroids, you may also be prone to develop shingles. For reasons yet unknown, the Caucasian race appears to have a higher incidence of shingles than other races. Your chest will be most affected by shingles. A nerve coming off of your brain that distributes branches to your face called the trigeminal nerve is the next most common nerve affected. Next the nerves off of your neck (called the cranial nerves) are affected, followed by the nerves coming off of your spinal cord that go to your legs (called the lumbar nerves). As you can see, shingles can affect nerves all over your body. After you have been diagnosed with shingles, your doctor will probably treat you with an antiviral drug. Acyclovir, famciclovir, and valacyclovir can be used for the treatment of your viral infection. Antiviral medications are used to decrease the intensity and duration of your shingles and are used to prevent the chronic pain associated with post-herpetic neuralgia.

Be aware that you can still have the onset of post-herpetic neuralgia even after treatment with these antiviral agents. Pain associated with post-herpetic neuralgia can be described as aching, burning, or stabbing. The worst pain is pain that is triggered by light touch such as clothing, bathing, or lying on a mattress. Sometimes cold weather or cold water can worsen your pain. Post-herpetic neuralgia is a dreaded complication of shingles. If you develop shingles and if your pain lasts longer than six weeks after your skin lesions have disappeared, you may have developed post-herpetic neuralgia. Be aware that a certain proportion of individuals who develop post-herpetic neuralgia will improve over time with no treatment. If you have post-herpetic neuralgia, the chances are that you will have improved by 12 months. Approximately 30 percent of individuals who develop post-herpetic neuralgia still complain of pain after one year. Two percent of individuals who suffer from post-herpetic neuralgia will have pain longer than five years.

If your pain is moderate, a mild analgesic such as Ultracet (tramadol) or a mild narcotic such as

Darvocet or Tylenol with codeine may suffice for the management of your pain. If your pain becomes excruciating, these medications will not provide you with any significant pain relief. At this time, you may require more potent opioid medication such as Percocet . If these stronger narcotic drugs do not provide you with relief, you may require the administration of a strong opioid medication such as morphine. If you develop post-herpetic neuralgia, avoid stressful situations that may worsen your pain. Avoid situations that cause you significant anxiety and/or depression. If you live in a cold environment, dress warmly.

In addition to antiviral agents, your doctor may prescribe steroids. Lotions, different types of patches, nonsteroidal anti-inflammatory drugs, antidepressants, and muscle relaxants may all be needed to control your pain. You may even need injections of numbing medicines into your nerves. Placement of local anesthetics around your sympathetic nerves may be of benefit in reducing your pain, especially if the injection is done soon after the onset of your pain. Topical agents are frequently used to treat shingles pain. These agents accelerate the healing of your skin and can decrease the pain associated with the shingles virus. However, topical anesthetics administered at the time that you develop shingles will not affect the development of post-herpetic neuralgia. Compresses or Burrow's solution or calamine lotion placed directly over your painful site can decrease the pain associated with acute herpes zoster.

A patch has been developed for the treatment of shingles. This patch called the Lidoderm patch has proven to be extremely useful in the management of shingles and post-herpetic neuralgia pain. A local anesthetic called lidocaine is placed within a patch system. The lidocaine is placed within an adhesive. The adhesive binds to your skin. Another type of transdermal (skin) drug-delivery system is a clonidine transdermal patch. This is placed over the area of your maximal pain. This drug is a drug that controls an individual's blood pressure. Tricyclic antidepressants are frequently used for the management of pain associated with post-herpetic neuralgia. In fact, tricyclic antidepressants are used to treat a variety of chronic pain syndromes. The exact mechanism by which these drugs decrease your pain is unknown. If narcotics are to be used, mild narcotics (Tramadol) should be initiated, as previously stated. Morphine is commonly used for severe pain. Baclofen, Amantadine, and Elavil can decrease your burning pain associated with post-herpetic neuralgia while anticonvulsant medications can lessen your sharp, shooting pain. Another topical drug that is sometimes used is capsaicin cream. It can be purchased over the counter and can also be purchased by prescription at a higher concentration. A newer anticonvulsant drug called Lyrica (pregabilin) is very effective in decreasing your pain.

Sometimes your doctor may want to put numbing medicine mixed with a steroid around your affected nerve. If you are experiencing pain in your chest wall, for example, your doctor may place an injection into the nerve that provides sensation to your chest.

This nerve is called the intercostal nerve. The type of nerve block used to treat your pain depends on the type of pain that you have. The pain associated with post-herpetic neuralgia can be somatic, sympathetic, or central. The somatic pain follows a certain nerve that is affected. Sympathetic pain can decrease the blood flow to your tissues and causes you to have a burning pain. Central pain is a result of rewiring of your central nervous system. For this type of pain, you need a different type of block. Sympathetic nerve blocks, if done early, can relieve pain associated with shingles and can also decrease the incidence of developing post-herpetic neuralgia. To be effective, they should be performed within the first two months after the onset of your symptoms. Stellate ganglion blocks are used for pain in your head, neck, and arms. Thoracic epidural blocks are used for pain in your mid back and chest wall, whereas lumbar sympathetic blocks are used for the management of post-herpetic neuralgia pain in your lower extremities. The purpose of nerve blocks is to interrupt your pain impulses and to facilitate therapy and to help you increase your daily-living activities. Nerve blocks should be used if your pain is becoming too severe and cannot be controlled by non-narcotic medications.

Occasionally a dorsal column stimulator can be placed in your epidural space to manage your pain. The dorsal column stimulator is essentially an epidural catheter that has electrodes on it. The number of electrodes that are used depends on the pattern of your pain. The dorsal column stimulator is placed within your body on a trial basis. The catheter is placed on an out-patient basis with x-ray. The end of the catheter attaches to a battery pack which can be placed under your skin. How the dorsal column stimulator actually works is debated. It is believed that the electrical interference with ascending pathways may be the mechanism for decreasing your pain impulse transmission. The use of this device has been demonstrated to be effective for the management of post-herpetic neuralgic pain that is refractory to all other modalities. The goal of the stimulation is to decrease your pain by at least 50 percent. If you do obtain adequate pain relief, the stimulator is implanted permanently surgically.

## 26. RSD (Reflex Sympathetic Dystrophy)

Reflex sympathetic dystrophy (RSD) affects one or more of your arms or legs but also can affect your face following a tooth extraction. Reflex sympathetic dystrophy is now called the Complex Regional Pain Syndrome (CRPS). Reflex sympathetic dystrophy is serious, painful, and potentially disabling. Pain associated with this entity is throbbing, burning, or aching. You can have pain just to light touch (alodynia). You can have swelling of one or more of your extremities as well as either warmth or coldness depending on the phase of your RSD and sweating also occurs on the palms of your hands or the soles of your feet. Your hair may grow faster on the extremity with RSD at first, only to progress to loss of hair on your arm or leg. Your extremity will sweat if you have RSD. It can turn color. The nails in your affected limb can grow faster on the extremity that suffers from reflex sympathetic dystrophy.

Reflex sympathetic dystrophy usually occurs following an injury. However, a heart attack or stroke can also trigger reflex sympathetic dystrophy. It can be seen in the knee as well as in the shoulder. Reflex sympathetic dystrophy occurs in 40 percent of the cases followed an injury to a muscle or a nerve. Simple bruises or sprains can also trigger reflex sympathetic dystrophy. Fractures account for 25 percent of reflex sympathetic dystrophy cases. Twenty percent of the RSD patients are postoperative on an arm or leg, whereas 12 percent occurred after a heart attack. Three percent of cases occur after a stroke. Approximately 37 percent of patients in a previous study had emotional disturbances at the time of the onset of the reflex sympathetic dystrophy.

It was once thought that reflex sympathetic dystrophy was caused by an emotional problem. Many people do not suffer from emotional problems at the time of the onset of reflex sympathetic dystrophy. Treatment usually consists of oral medications as well as injection therapy by an anesthesiologist using local anesthetics. Steroids may also be used effectively to treat RSD. If you sustained actual nerve damage, your reflex sympathetic dystrophy is called causalgia or complex regional pain syndrome II. Complex regional pain syndrome I does not have a nerve injury associated with it.

Reflex sympathetic dystrophy is a syndrome that consists of burning pain, pain to touch over the skin of the injured extremity, shiny skin, and skin that has different colors consisting of either redness or a blue cyanotic color. Blue or cyanotic discoloration usually occurs when skin or other tissues do not get enough blood and oxygen. With this disease, the pain in your extremity is out of proportion to your injury. It was originally hypothesized that if your sympathetic nervous system became hyperactive, this hyperactivity caused of reflex sympathetic dystrophy. Your sympathetic nervous system is one component of your autonomic nervous system. The other component is called the parasympathetic nervous system. Your autonomic nervous system regulates your circulation and your breathing as well as your stomach and bladder functions. You have no control over your autonomic nervous system. Your sympathetic nervous system sends sympathetic nerve fibers to the blood vessels in your head and neck as well as to your skin, muscles and sweat glands in your arms and legs. Your hands and feet can sweat profusely if you have reflex sympathetic dystrophy and the hair on your arms and legs can grow faster or fall out. Your sympathetic nerve fibers can also restrict circulation in certain areas of your body. Sometimes if your doctor blocks your sympathetic nerve pathways with a numbing medicine, you can have some relief of your reflex sympathetic dystrophy. The treatment of reflex sympathetic dystrophy includes weekly repetitive sympathetic blocks up to 5 or 6 or removal of the sympathetic nerves, either surgically or by chemicals such as phenol or by intense heat. Sympathetic blocks involve placing a local anesthetic about the bundles of nerves that exist outside of your central nervous system. These nerve bundles that are called ganglia are in your neck as well as your lower back. The ganglion in your neck influences your arm pain- while your ganglion in your lower back influences RSD pain in your leg.

For you to be diagnosed with RSD, you should have the following: An initiating traumatic event to your body (e.g. bone fracture), an onset of spontaneous pain, excruciating pain to light touch (allodynia) as well as pain from a noxious stimulus that lasts longer than expected. Your pain must be global and not just confined to a specific area. For example, if you have injured your hand, you may have an injury to one of the nerves in your hand. Your ulnar nerve will give you pain or numbness in your last two fingers of your hand if this nerve is affected. This is the definition of a neuritis that means inflammation of a nerve. This is not RSD. This is an example of neuralgia. RSD means that the whole hand (global) is painful and not just in the distribution of one nerve. Other signs of reflex sympathetic dystrophy include evidence of swelling of your extremity, an increase or a decrease in your skin blood flow noted by imaging as well as alterations in the color of your skin and sweating. Cold applications to your skin can worsen your pain. Movement of your joints can also cause pain if you have RSD. You skin may be shiny. Your nails should grow faster on the side of the reflex sympathetic dystrophy. At first your hair will grow faster on the side of your reflex sympathetic dystrophy but eventually your hair pattern will decrease and you may even lose hair in this area.

RSD must be treated immediately once it has been diagnosed. If you have any of these symptoms mentioned in this chapter, notify your doctor. A three-phase bone scan can be useful in diagnosing reflex sympathetic dystrophy. This imagery is related to the distribution of a radioactive isotope throughout the body, and a nuclear medicine doctor will examine the distribution of the radioactive isotope in the affected extremity. The distribution of the radioactive isotope is dependent upon blood flow as well as the activity of the bone. In early RSD, Phase I, you will have increased blood flow and after 3 months your blood flow will be decreased. If your three-phase bone scan is negative, this does not mean that you do not have reflex sympathetic dystrophy. A three-phase bone scan may be effective for staging the early or late forms of RSD. Magnetic resonance imaging (MRI) can also aid in the diagnosis of RSD by identifying swelling in the center of your bone. This bone marrow edema is characteristic of complex regional pain syndrome. This study is more reliable than a three-phase bone scanning or plain X-ray exams.

Contact and infrared thermography have both been used for the diagnosis of reflex sympathetic dystrophy, but the problem with thermography is that it can be influenced not only by skin blood flow but also by the temperature of the room environment as well as by your muscle and your deep tissue metabolism. A new method called laser Doppler imaging has been shown to be effective for the diagnosis of complex regional pain syndrome. The laser Doppler is important because the results of this study are influenced by your skin blood flow. Your skin blood flow is under the control of your autonomic nervous system. As your RSD progresses, the blood vessels to your extremity will decrease in caliber. They go from their enlarged diameter to a normal appearing diameter. This is phase II. You will have some swelling as well at this time and global pain about your extremity and sweating of your extremity as your sympathetic nervous system becomes overactive. This phase can progress on to phase III. During phase III, your blood vessels become extremely small and you have decreased blood flow to your hand, foot, or your affected extremity. This will cause your skin to become cold. By this time, you will notice that your skin has become shiny and that the sweating in your hand or foot may have increased. A three-phase bone scan at this time can detect a significant decrease in your blood flow to your extremity. Your treating doctor should try and prevent you from progressing through these phases by being aggressive in his or her treatment.

Clonidine, which is frequently prescribed as a patch over your skin, can also be administered into your epidural space for the control of your pain as well. Baclofen or a snail toxin toenails on the affected extremity can become thick and clubbed. The frequency of reflex sympathetic dystrophy shows a peak incidence of this entity around 50 years of age. However, you must be aware that both children and elderly individuals can develop RSD. RSD can be refractive to treatment with sympathetic blockade. This type of RSD is called sympathetically independent pain. RSD related pain that responds to sympathetic blockade is classified as sympathetically maintained pain. Sympathetically maintained pain usually has a decrease in your pain component following a sympathetic block. The onset of reflex sympathetic dystrophy can occur at any time following a traumatic event ranging from days to months.

The exact cause of reflex sympathetic dystrophy is unknown. If you have had a nerve injury where your nerve was cut, your nerve endings will attempt to grow together. The nerve endings will sprout small nerve fibers. Sometimes as your nerves attempt to grow together, the area where they come together can be extremely painful. Where the nerve endings come together can cause an extremely painful area called a neuroma. This neuroma is sensitive to the chemicals released by your sympathetic nervous system. Females are more vulnerable to sympathetically mediated pain than males. The chemicals that are involved that cause you to have reflex sympathetic dystrophy are potentially affected by your sex hormones. It is believed that your hormone status at the time of your trauma is important for the development of the pain associated with reflex sympathetic dystrophy. The effects of reflex sympathetic dystrophy on the central processing in your central nervous system may be the basis for the spread of reflex sympathetic dystrophy to your other extremities. Many recommendations for the treatment of reflex sympathetic dystrophy exist. Because there are so many different treatments proposed, you should be aware that no single treatment is superior to the others. Remember that no treatment for complex regional pain syndrome is consistently successful. It is known that early recognition and active treatment of the complex regional pain syndrome improves your outcome. For example, injections of local anesthetics about your sympathetic nervous system can alleviate your symptoms of reflex sympathetic dystrophy for weeks to months. In some instances the relief may be permanent. These types of injections must be done early following the onset of your symptoms of reflex sympathetic dystrophy. The injections can be done in your stellate ganglion, which provides sympathetic fibers to your arms, or the injections can be done in the lumbar sympathetic ganglion, which supplies sympathetic fibers to your legs and feet.

    A clonidine patch can be used to decrease your pain. This patch is usually used to treat high blood pressure. However, the patch does decrease the sympathetic nervous system chemicals that can be released if you have reflex sympathetic dystrophy. The patch is usually worn for one week before it is changed. Steroids administered by mouth are effective for the treatment of reflex sympathetic dystrophy. Steroids will decrease inflammation caused by prostaglandins. If your pain is severe, your doctor will probably prescribe a narcotic drug for you. Depending on the severity of your pain, your doctor will prescribe a mild narcotic such as Darvocet (propoxyphene) or a stronger narcotic such as methadone. Anticonvulsive medications can be helpful in decreasing your pain. Gabapentin (Neurontin) is frequently used now for the treatment of pain associated with your complex regional pain syndrome.

    Narcotic medications administered into your spinal fluid can help decrease your pain. Antidepressant medications such as amitriptyline have also been shown to be effective. Amitriptyline increases certain chemicals in your central nervous system that are helpful in decreasing the amount of pain that reaches your brain. Implantation of an electrical spinal wire attached to a battery into your epidural space can also provide you with significant pain relief. This apparatus is called a dorsal column stimulator. Psychological intervention is also helpful; because of the severity of the pain associated with reflex sympathetic dystrophy, you can develop fear, anxiety, and depression. Psychological intervention including the use of biofeedback and sometimes hypnosis can successfully be used to treat your pain.

    Whatever treatment is chosen to treat RSD, the most important consideration is the rapid diagnosis and institution of treatment to prevent this disease from becoming disabling.

# 27. VASCULAR DISEASE

Vascular diseases have tendencies to obstruct blood flow to areas throughout your body. For example, patients with Raynaud's disease have complaints of burning pain, numbness and swelling in their fingers, toes or hands or feet on both arms. Raynaud's phenomenon usually involves one hand and is related to some lesion that compresses arteries to your hands. Raynaud's disease affects both hands while Raynaud's phenomenon can affect one hand. Diseases that contribute to Raynaud's disease or phenomena include obstructive arterial disorders, vascular disorders, and scleroderma. Drug intoxications as well as some cancers and neurological entities can cause Raynaud's disease. Raynaud's disease is a vascular pain. Raynaud's disease pain can last a few minutes to hours. The average length of attack is 5 minutes to 60 minutes.

Raynaud's disease is a disorder of blood flow to your fingers, toes, nose, ears, and sometimes your tongue. When you have symptoms, you will suddenly experience a decrease in your blood flow to these areas. You will have color changes of your skin, especially on your fingers and toes, with exposure to cold or emotional stress. Cold exposure to your face can also cause changes in your fingers and toes. Many people use the term Raynaud's disease to include Raynaud's phenomena. This disease is classified as one of two types: primary and secondary. Secondary Raynaud's disease is also called Raynaud's phenomena. Primary Raynaud's disease has no underlying medical problem and is mild and causes fewer complications than secondary Raynaud's disease. Approximately 50 percent of people diagnosed with Raynaud's disease are primary Raynaud's disease and 50 percent are Raynaud's phenomena. Women are five times more likely than men to develop primary Raynaud's disease. Most patients develop Raynaud's disease before age 40. Be aware that 30 percent of individuals with primary Raynaud's disease progress to secondary Raynaud's disease. Approximately 15 percent of individuals with primary Raynaud's disease do improve. The secondary Raynaud's disease or Raynaud's phenomena is essentially the same as primary Raynaud's disease but secondary Raynaud's disease occurs in individuals who have predisposing factors.

You need to know that there are three phases of Raynaud's disease. When you are first exposed to cold, your small arteries contract and your fingers, toes, ears, or the tip of your nose and tongue become pale and white. This observation occurs because you are deprived of blood. Remember if you have an increased blood flow to your tissues, the tissue will appear red. After your oxygen is deprived, your blood vessels will expand. It is the veins that expand most. The veins carry blood that has minimal or no oxygen. This will give your blood a bluish tint. The area of the low-oxygen-carrying blood will appear blue. The area also feels cold to touch. When your arteries begin to dilate, the blood flow is increased. Oxygen is increased and your tissue color will appear normal. Primary Raynaud's disease can be later classified as a secondary Raynaud's disease after a predisposing underlying disease has been diagnosed. This observation is seen in 30 percent of patients. A secondary type of Raynaud's disease is more complicated and severe. This type of Raynaud's disease is more likely to worsen. Diseases that can predispose you to secondary Raynaud's disease include scleroderma, SLE, rheumatoid arthritis, and polio. For some reason, herniated discs and spinal cord tumors as well as cerebrovascular accidents and polio can progress to Raynaud's disease. Vascular pain in general can be divided into three categories: Arterial pain, pain due to dysfunction of the capillaries in your tissue and pain related to pathology of your veins. You can have obstruction of both your arteries and veins of your limbs. When this happens you have what is called Burger's disease. Swelling of the small arteries and veins in your extremities causes this disease. The painful symptoms that you note are a result again of decreased oxygen flow to your tissues.

When your blood supply to a part of your body is decreased, which happens in Burger's disease, your oxygen to your tissue is significantly decreased. You will develop pain in the calves of your legs. If the oxygen deficit is extremely low, your nerves to your legs will suffer injury. This nerve injury will cause you pain as well as lack of oxygen to your extremity muscles. If your pain is severe, you may not experience relief with rest. If your tissues are deprived of oxygen for a long time, you can develop ulcerations in your skin and also develop gangrene. Another problem with your blood vessels that can cause you to have pain is Takayasu's syndrome. This syndrome is due to inflammation or swelling of your small arteries of the upper part of your body, including your eyes. It occurs more in young girls as well as young women. More than 60 percent of individuals complain of weakness and fever as well as joint pain and pain in the upper extremities. When this pain occurs, you will soon develop the pain about the arteries that are inflamed. This disease can progress to even cause you to have angina pectoris. If this angina pectoris progresses, you may have a heart attack as well.

Temporal arteritis is another inflammation of the large arteries, especially around your temples. Inflammation of one or both of these arteries can cause you to have significant headaches. It can also involve other branches of your carotid artery. Temporal arteritis occurs usually if you are over 55 years of age. Temporal arteritis is more common in women than in men. Occasionally if you have temporal arteritis you will have headaches that are occasionally unbearable. Your headache will begin over your involved arteries. As stated, the pain mostly begins about your temples. However, this disease can also affect your occipital arteries. These are the arteries that are toward the back of your head and approximate an area where the back of your skull meets your neck. You may have tenderness to touch over the swollen and inflamed arteries. The areas around your inflamed arteries are extremely sensitive to firm touch. You may even have decreased blood flow to your jaw muscles. Therefore, when you chew you may have significant pain in your jaw muscles. Temporal arteritis can affect arteries in multiple locations throughout your body. You may develop a flulike syndrome with generalized muscle pain as well as fever and weakness. The muscle pain can progress and involve your neck, shoulders, and pelvis as well as your legs. The arteries are usually affected on both sides of your body.

Erythemalgia is a syndrome that can affect both your arms and your legs. The temperature in your extremities will be elevated and you will have redness in either your arms or legs. Along with the change in color, you will have burning pain as well as tingling in your extremities. Sometimes you will experience swelling in your hands and feet. Usually this disease affects your legs. However, it can also affect your arms. This entity is usually seen if you are exposed to an increased temperature. When you experience the pain, it can last for a few minutes up to hours. This type of pain in this syndrome can be associated with diabetes.

Sickle cell disease affects the arteries throughout your body. This pain can be severe. The sickling cells can stop blood flow to your blood vessels. As a result, you have generalized lack of oxygen to all of your tissues and have severe pain. Sickle cell disease is inherited. Sickle cell disease is more prevalent in African Americans or individuals of Mediterrean decent. In Africa, the sickle cell gene gave advantage to individuals because it would resist infection caused by malaria. This is the reason why the disease is prevalent in populations of African descent. The deposition of sickled cells within your arteries decreases blood flow to your tissues. This causes a painful crisis to the majority of your organs. If you have sickle cell disease and if you have a painful crisis, you will note the development of severe pain. The frequency of the pain occurs most in the third and fourth decades. Cold and infection can induce you to have a sickle cell crisis. Furthermore, dehydration and alcohol consumption can cause you to have a crisis as well as exposure to low-oxygen tension. You can have pain in different parts of your body. Chest pain can occur. This is usually accompanied by a fever. You back, legs, and stomach may also develop significant pain. If you have pain in your abdomen, this pain can mimic appendicitis. The sickle cell related pain can last from hours to even weeks. You can have a gradual or sudden onset of pain. You can have decreased blood flow to your bone. This will cause some tissue death in your bone. You can have pain in your joints as well as swelling. This pain is severe enough to cause you to experience depression.

The initial treatment of this disease is usually the administration of either steroids or nonsteroidal anti-inflammatory drugs. If your pain is severe, your doctor may prescribe narcotic medications until your crisis subsides. If you have infection as a cause of your sickle cell crisis, you may require antibiotics. Because of the depression associated with this entity, you may need to have a psychological evaluation as well as the administration of antidepressant drugs. Sometimes narcotic medications are necessary for pain control.

Scleroderma also affects your skin. By definition, it is called "hard skin." It is uncommon. Scleroderma is classified according to the degree of your skin thickening. Scleroderma is most common in adults. However, it can be seen in children. The hallmarks of scleroderma are light skin and Raynaud's phenomena. Scleroderma is a generalized disorder of the small arteries as well as the connective tissue around your arteries. Not only can your gastrointestinal tract be affected but also your lungs, your heart, and your kidneys. Most all patients who have scleroderma have Raynaud's disease. Patients with scleroderma can have pallor of the digits following cold exposure or emotional stress. Your fingers and toes can turn blue followed by redness in addition to burning pain and tingling.

This disease can be severe and devastating. You can get gangrene in your fingers and toes and end up with an amputation. Swelling can be seen over your hands and feet. Over time, thinning of your skin can occur. The thinning of your skin is easily noted over joints. Usually scleroderma begins before age 40 and is more common in females. Approximately 80 percent of scleroderma patients are females. Scleroderma can affect your kidneys and may cause you to have kidney failure. Scleroderma can also affect your heart and cause heart arrhythmias and palpations.. You may need an echocardiograph if you have chest pain. This test can reveal some thickening around the outer wall of your heart. You will have muscle pain as well as joint pain if you have scleroderma. You will have stiffness in the morning. Systemic lupus erythematosus is a disease of unknown cause. It can also be associated with Raynaud's disease.

Systemic lupus erythematosus (SLE) is caused by your body's production of antibodies that injure the tissues of some of your organs in your body. The symptoms can come and go. You may have a rash develop on your face. However, SLE can be life threatening if it involves your internal organs. SLE can cause you to have failure of your kidneys or hemorrhage as well as a pulmonary disease. Dermatomyositis is an inflammatory disease that can affect your muscles. You will have muscle pain and tenderness. A rash usually accompanies this disease. The rash occurs on your upper eyelids. You may have some swelling around your eyes as well. You can have redness about the knuckles of your fingers. This disease can affect almost any organ system in your body. You can have involvement of the muscles of your fingers and toes. The muscles in your legs can become weak. This disease can be caused by an abnormality in your immune system. The diagnosis of this disease can be done by taking samples of your muscle.

Polyarteritis nodosa is caused by inflammation or swelling of the walls of your blood vessels. This disease can affect blood vessels of any size as well as in any location. It usually occurs between ages 40 and 50. Men are affected more than women. Your kidneys can be affected. If the disease progresses, you can develop kidney failure. This disease can affect your arteries going to your heart and can cause you to have a heart attack. It may cause abdominal pain and bleeding. This disease can affect your nervous system as well. It can cause you to have weakness as well as loss of sensation. As stated previously, it can be associated with rheumatoid arthritis.

## 28. CANCER PAIN

Cancer pain is usually not evident until the cancer growth has become far advanced. Most non-solid tumors cause minimal pain while solid tumors like prostate cancer can cause significant pain. If you have myeloma, you will have a malignant formation of your plasma cells. Plasma cells are antibody-producing cells found in bone forming tissue as well as in your lungs and your abdomen. This increase in your plasma cells can affect your organs and cause you to have painful symptoms. Usually bone pain is the most common pain noted involving multiple myeloma. The bone pain associated with this entity involves primarily the back. If you have multiple myeloma, your pain is usually worse at night and is made worse by movement. This disease can destroy your bone. With significant destruction of your bone, your bone can collapse. If the bones in your spine collapse, the collapsed bone can injure your spinal cord. With injury to your spinal cord, you can lose control of your bowel and your bladder and even become paralyzed. Oncologists sometimes request the help of a pain medicine specialist to help manage their patient's cancer pain. You should now be aware that any type of pathology that will decrease the blood flow to your tissue can cause you to have significant pain.

Lung cancer is common in the United States. Lung Cancer is a disease that begins in the tissue of the lungs. The lungs are sponge-like organs that are part of the respiratory system. During breathing, air enters the mouth or nasal passage and travels down the trachea. The trachea splits into two sets of bronchial tubes that lead to the left and right lung. The bronchi branch off into smaller and smaller tubes that eventually end in small balloon-like sacs known as alveoli. The alveoli are where oxygen is taken up by your body and carbon dioxide is removed. The vast majority of lung cancer cases fall into one of two different categories: Non-Small Cell Lung Cancer is the most common type of lung cancer, making up nearly 80% of all cases. This type of lung cancer grows and spreads more slowly than small cell lung cancer. Small Cell Lung Cancer makes up nearly 20% of all lung cancer cases. It is associated with cancer cells smaller than most other cancer cells. These cells may be small, but they can rapidly reproduce to form large tumors. Their size and quick rate of reproduction allows them to spread to the lymph nodes and to other organs of the body. Cigarette smoking causes this type of cancer.

Colon cancer is another common cancer that you need to be aware of. The colon is the part of your body where the waste material is stored. The rectum is the end of the colon adjacent to the anus. Together, they form a long, muscular tube called the large intestine (also known as the large bowel). Tumors of the colon and rectum are growths arising from the inner wall of the large intestine. Benign tumors of the large intestine are called polyps. Malignant tumors of the large intestine are called cancers. Cancer of the colon and rectum (also referred to as colorectal cancer) can invade and damage adjacent tissues and organs. Cancer cells can also break away and spread to other parts of the body (such as your liver and lung. Factors that increase a person's risk of colorectal cancer include high fat intake, a family history of colorectal cancer and polyps, the presence of polyps in the large intestine, and chronic ulcerative colitis. Symptoms of colon cancer are usually nonspecific. They include: fatigue, weakness, and shortness of breath, change in bowel habits, bloody stools, diarrhea and/ or constipation, blood in your stool, weight loss, abdominal pain or cramps. If colon cancer is suspected a barium enema x ray or a colonoscopy will be done. Surgery is the most common treatment for cancer of the rectum and colon. If the cancer has spread you may also require chemotherapy. If your cancer is limited to your rectum, you may be treated with radiation therapy.

Some cancers can be gender specific. For example, if you are a female, you can develop cancer of your breasts, cervix, uterus, or ovary. If you are male, you can develop cancer of your testicles, prostate gland or breast. Cancer-related pain can be excruciating in some cases. Various treatment methods and therapies are available to help relieve your pain if it is caused by a cancer. Breast cancer is the most common malignancy in women in the United States. Approximately 182,000 women develop breast cancer and more than 46,000 die with it. It occurs in one in eight women. Approximately two thirds of cases occur after menopause. Fifteen percent of cases occur before the age of 40. Screening for female cancers is very important. The majority of women detect their own breast cancer. You should have a breast examination by your doctor at the time of your regular physical examination if you are over age 40. Mammography is recommended every 1 to 2 years if you are older than 40 years of age.

If you have a history of breast cancer, you should have a mammogram yearly. If you are over 40 and have a family history of breast cancer, you should also have a mammogram every year. The survival rate is lower if your cancer is detected by a mammogram as opposed to palpation. Breast cancer is usually painless and presents with a palpable mass in a postmenopausal woman. If it had associated pain, the diagnosis would be earlier diagnosed. You should perform routine self-examinations as your cancer can be diagnosed early as opposed to waiting for your doctor or mammogram to make the diagnosis. An accurate diagnosis of breast cancer requires a needle aspiration, a percutaneous needle biopsy, or an incisional (surgical) biopsy. A biopsy should be done on every suspicious breast mass. You must have a chest x-ray to see if your breast cancer may have spread to your lungs, ribs, or spine. A bone scan may also be required to see if your breast cancer has spread to your bones. If you have breast cancer, your doctor will want to get a CAT scan of your abdomen to see if the cancer has affected your liver as well. Risks for breast cancer include increasing age, a family history of breast cancer, previous cancer in one breast, early menstruation (meaning before age 12), late menopause (meaning after age 52), a history of having no children, obesity, a high fat diet, alcohol use, and a family history of cancer of the ovary, uterus, or colon.

A pathologist will stage your cancer. Staging determines the severity of your cancer. A 0 stage cancer is confined to an area of your organ. A stage greater than III usually means that the cancer has spread beyond your involved organ. Your survival rate depends on the stage of the cancer. The stages are based on the severity of the cancer. The higher the stage correlates with a lower survival rate. If you have cancer in your breast that has not spread to your bones or other organs, your 5-year survival rate is greater than 95 percent. However, if your cancer has spread to other areas of your body, your 5-year survival rate is only 10 percent. If your cancer is only in your tissue, you may only need removal of that part of the tissue from your breast. If your breast cancer has spread to other areas of your body, you will most likely require a mastectomy (removal of your breast, radiation therapy, chemotherapy, as well as hormone therapy).

With respect to female cancer, cervical cancer accounts for approximately 2 to 3 percent of all cancers involving women in the United States. More than 15,000 cases of cervical cancer are diagnosed each year, and approximately 5,000 women die from this disease. Risk factors for developing carcinoma of the cervix include suppression of the immune system, a history of genital herpes or genital warts, multiple sexual partners, partners with penile warts or cancer, low economic status, intercourse before age 17, and cigarette smoking. Usually cancer of the cervix is painless. A Pap smear detects many cases of cervical cancer. If you have abnormal vaginal bleeding, vaginal discharge, or bleeding after intercourse, you may have advanced cervical cancer. Cancer from your cervix can spread and can cause you to experience lower back pain, leg pain, weight loss, or swelling in your legs. If you have an abnormal Pap smear, you will have a biopsy of your cervix. If the biopsy is unable to determine whether a suspicious-looking tissue is cancerous, you will have a greater portion of your cervix removed, which is called a cervical conization.

Standard therapy for uterine cancer is an abdominal hysterectomy with removal of both your ovaries. As with other cancers mentioned in this chapter, you should have a pelvic exam and Pap smear every three months for the first two years after treatment. Other tests should be done only if you have a recurrence of symptoms. If you do have recurrence of the cancer, a major surgical procedure will need to be done. Ovarian cancer develops in 1 in every 70 women. Approximately 1 percent of women die from this cancer. Approximately 24,000 cases of ovarian cancer are diagnosed in the United States each year. More than 13,000 women will die with ovarian cancer each year.

The incidence of cancer of the ovary is increased in women who have never been pregnant and is more prevalent in women who have had late onset of menopause or have been on a high-fat diet. If you are female and have a history of colon cancer or breast cancer, you are at a higher risk for developing ovarian cancer. If you are using oral contraceptives, have had more than one baby, and are breast-feeding, you will have a decreased risk of developing cancer of the ovaries. If someone in your family has a history of ovarian cancer, you are at an increased risk. If your cancer is confined to your ovary, you have a stage 1A cancer. You have a five-year survival rate of approximately 90 percent. If you have a stage IV ovarian tumor, the cancer has spread to your liver or lung or so forth. Your five-year survival rate is 5 percent. You can have abnormal uterine bleeding. If you are a postmenopausal female and if your doctor can palpate your ovary on a routine pelvic exam, this suggests that you may have an ovarian tumor. If you have ovarian cancer, you will have your ovaries removed as well as your uterus. You will also have surgical sampling of your lymph glands to see whether your cancer has spread to your lymph glands. Chemotherapy may be prescribed to your after surgery. Your prognosis is good if you are relatively young and if you have an early stage of the cancer and if you have a rapid rate of your ovarian tumor response to the therapy mentioned.

Males suffer from gender specific tumors as well. The testes secrete testosterone and estradiol, which are two hormones. Testicular cancer represents approximately 2 percent of all cancers in men. It is the second most common cancer in men between the ages of 20 and 34 years of age. These tumors usually manifest as an enlargement of the testicle. You may have pain and tenderness in your testicle. A male with a testicular tumor can have breast enlargement. Approximately 10 percent of these tumors will have distant spread of the cancer at the time of the diagnosis. These tumors are staged through measurement of certain chemical markers in the bloodstream as well as imaging studies or surgery. Some of these cancers are quite sensitive to radiation therapy. Other tumors that are confined to the testes are cured through removal of the testicle followed by radiation therapy. If your tumor has spread throughout your body, the disease is treated with both radiation therapy and chemotherapy. If your cancer is localized to your testicle, your 5-year survival rate approximates 100 percent. If your cancer has spread throughout your body, your survival rate drops to 20 percent.

Most men over 55 years of age may have an enlargement of their prostate gland. Almost two thirds of these men will have symptoms of prostatism. They will have decreased force of their urine stream and retention of their urine in their bladder after they urinate. Cancer symptoms may be without significant symptoms initially but as the cancer advances can become severe. Prostate cancer is the second most common tumor in men. Lung cancer is the most common. Approximately 200,000 new cases are diagnosed each year in the United States. Prostate cancer is more common among African Americans and men who have a family history of prostate cancer. The problem with prostate cancer is that it is usually painless and has no other symptoms that are seen with prostatism. Prostate cancer can be detected by routine digital examination or elevation of your prostate specific antigen (PSA). Sometimes if you have surgery to remove an enlarged prostate gland, cancer tissue can be found in your prostate gland. Your prostate cancer is usually testosterone sensitive. Your doctor will prescribe hormone therapy that will lower your testosterone in your bloodstream. This can be done through castration.

There is no reason why cancer pain cannot be controlled. There are multiple modalities now available to adequately control cancer pain. If you have been diagnosed with cancer, you face a wide range of psychological and physical problems throughout your cancer. You may have a fear of a painful death or disfigurement. One of the most feared consequences of cancer is pain. To treat your pain appropriately, a multidisciplinary approach may be necessary, including your oncologist, your psychologist or psychiatrist, and your pain-management doctor. Neuropathic pain causes you to experience symptoms that are sharp and electrical shock like. This type of pain can be controlled by antiseizure medications such as Neurontin or Lyrica. You can have pain that is severe and excessive for the extent of tissue damage that has occurred. This type of pain is called idiopathic and usually has a psychological pathology associated with it.

Anticonvulsant medications can relieve severe lancinating pain when your tumor affects one of your nerves. In case you are wondering why a seizure medication would be prescribed, it's because these medications are also pain medications. In the United States, about 5 percent of all anticonvulsant medications are prescribed for pain management. Nerve injury caused by cancer, chemotherapy, or radiation therapy is controlled with anticonvulsant medications. Nonsteroidal anti-inflammatory medications may relieve bone pain related to your cancer. Narcotics can relieve your cancer pain. Morphine is the standard of comparison for the rest of the narcotic analgesics. A sustained-release preparation is available called MS Contin releases the drug over 8 to 12 hours. Oxycontin also provides a release of oxycodone over 8-12 hours. Dilaudid is stronger than morphine, but it has a shorter duration of action than morphine. Methadone is another drug that can be prescribed for cancer pain. It is very effective when given in a pill form. Another drug more potent than morphine is Levo-Dromoran. It is stronger than morphine. Fentanyl is a potent drug that is more potent than the drugs mentioned. A transdermal fentanyl patch gives you a continuous dose of fentanyl. Cancer pain can be successfully treated. In order to do so, a timely and accurate diagnosis must be done. This is one of many reasons why you should have a routine physical examination by your doctor.

# 29. CHEST PAIN

Chest pain can be a frightful experience, as you probably know. Heart related pain requires immediate attention. However, not every chest pain is related to heart pathology. You have many structures in your chest that can be a cause of your chest pain. Shingles that is discussed in another chapter in this book can cause some chest pain. Even though minor medical conditions can cause you to have chest pain, if you are having a heart attack, it can be potentially fatal. For this reason, any chest pain should not be taken lightly. Chest pain is difficult to diagnose. Chest pain is vague. There are many structures in your chest cavity. You have two lungs, a diaphragm, a heart and a larynx and an esophagus. Furthermore, these organs have wrappers around them. The organs are wrapped by a peritoneum. The peritoneum contains many pain fibers. If your peritoneum becomes inflamed you may experience chest pain.

The heart's function is to pump blood. The right side of the heart pumps blood to the lungs, where oxygen is added to the blood and carbon dioxide is removed from it. The left side pumps blood to the rest of the body, where oxygen and nutrients are delivered to tissues and waste products are transferred to the blood for removal by other organs. With respect to the chest pain example presented at the beginning of this chapter you need to realize that as people age, the heart tends to enlarge slightly, developing thicker walls and slightly larger chambers. These changes are usually not work related. The increase in heart size is mainly due to an increase in the size of individual heart muscle cells. During rest, the older heart function in almost the same way as a younger heart except the heart rate in the older individual is slightly lower. However, during exercise, the older heart cannot increase the amount of blood pumped out as much as a younger heart. The walls of the arteries and arterioles become thicker as you age, and the space within the arteries expands slightly. Elastic tissue within the walls of the arteries and arterioles is lost. Together, these changes make your blood the vessels stiffer.

Because arteries and arterioles become less elastic as you get older, they cannot relax as quickly during the pumping of the heart. As a result, blood pressure increases in the older individual more when the heart contracts. High blood pressure during systole with normal blood pressure during diastole is very common among older people and this disorder is called isolated systolic hypertension. Many of the effects of aging on the heart and blood vessels can be reduced by regular exercise. Exercise helps you maintain cardiovascular fitness as well as muscular fitness. Exercise is beneficial regardless of the age at which it is initiated. The arteries can become clogged over time. If one of your arteries that supplies blood to your heart muscle is deprived of oxygen, you will experience chest pain (angina). If the lumen of your artery is completely obliterated then your heart muscle can become damaged causing you to have a heart attack (myocardial infarction). These changes occurred over time. Angina is pain in the center of your chest. Usually rest relieves angina. Anginal chest pain in men may spread to the jaws and arms. Pain that radiates from the left side of the chest into the left arm is especially characteristic of anginal pain in men. In women on the other hand, a decrease in oxygen to the heart muscle for some reason, causes anginal pain and pressure in the center of the chest accompanied by pain in the neck or arms. Angina or heart pain occurs when the demand for blood by the heart muscle exceeds the oxygen supply of the arteries. This why exercise like shoveling snow can cause angina.

A myocardial infarction (heart attack) or death of a segment of your heart muscle occurs following interruption of the blood supply to the heart muscle. This is more severe than angina. A heart attack can cause sudden severe chest pain. There is a danger that your heart could go into an irregular heartbeat called an arrhythmia. If you have a severe arrhythmia, your heart can stop, which is referred to as a cardiac arrest. If you have interruption of the blood flow going to your heart, you can have irreversible injury to your heart muscle. This injury usually begins within 20 minutes from the time of the loss of blood flow to your heart muscle. Therefore, if you think that you are having a heart attack, contact your local emergency room or your doctor. If your pain is severe, go directly to your emergency room by ambulance. Angina pectoris is chest pain that results from decreased oxygen supply to your heart muscle. Angina pectoris is usually pain under your breastbone. You may perceive discomfort instead of pain or pressure. The pain, if it is present or the pressure can radiate to your neck or arm that is usually your left arm. Shortness of breath may also be reported. Angina pectoris is usually elicited by physical exertion. Occasionally psychological stress can cause you to have angina pectoris. If you are worried about an impending job interview for example, you could develop angina. Exposure to cold air can cause angina. Angina comes on quickly and can last for up to 15 minutes. It usually resolves with rest or with nitroglycerin.

Coronary artery disease can be a cause of angina. Over time coronary artery disease can also cause you to have a heart attack (myocardial infarction). Lifestyle changes such as diet, exercise, and stopping smoking tobacco can decrease the incidence of coronary artery disease. Atherosclerosis is a build-up of fat and other materials in the walls of arteries that causes them to become narrowed. This entity is caused by many factors. If you are hypertensive and have an elevated cholesterol and smoke, you are at a higher risk for developing atherosclerosis. When you have a deposit of fat and calcium in your blood vessels, your heart will still pump blood through these vessels. It takes a decrease in the diameter of your blood vessels by approximately 70 percent to decrease your blood flow. Smoking is an important factor that can cause you to be at a high risk for developing coronary artery disease. When you smoke tobacco, the nicotine in the tobacco causes your coronary arteries to decrease in caliber. This action decreases blood flow to your heart muscles that decreases oxygen to your heart muscles. A decreased in heart muscle oxygen can cause a heart attack.

A high cholesterol blood level can increase your risk of developing coronary artery disease. If you have high levels of low-density lipoprotein cholesterol, you have an elevated chance of developing coronary heart disease. If your cholesterol is elevated, your doctor will help you reduce your cholesterol with both diet and with pharmacologic management. You must monitor your diet for fat intake. Cocaine can also contribute to heart disease. Cocaine use has become more and more prevalent in the United States. However, cocaine use can make the arteries in your heart to go into spasm. Cocaine can accelerate the deposition of fat and calcium in your blood vessels, which can cause you to have angina as well as a heart attack. You will develop chest pain when your heart oxygen demand exceeds the supply of oxygen that your blood vessels are delivering to your heart. If your heart begins beating faster, the increase in oxygen demand is met by an increased blood flow in your arteries about your heart. The small arteries around your heart muscle will increase their diameter to provide your heart with more oxygenated blood. If your vessels cannot dilate, your heart will not receive enough oxygen and you will experience pain in your chest. Fat and calcium within your heart vessels will restrict the amount of blood that goes to your heart.

According to the American Heart Association, approximately 6.3 million men and 6.6 million women in the United States have heart attacks. In the year 2000, more than 500,000 people died from heart disease. Different types of angina have been described. Stable angina is angina that is chronic and is usually caused by physical activity or emotional stress. Stable angina is usually heart-related pain relieved by rest or nitroglycerin. Unstable angina, on the other hand, can increase with rest. Other types of unstable angina can occur at low activity levels. Unstable angina may not be responsive to nitroglycerin. Sometimes you can develop spasms of your arteries that supply your heart muscle. This type of spasm is called Pinzmetal's angina and can be relieved frequently with nitroglycerin.

Stable angina is a term used to describe pain that is predictably caused by narrowing of your coronary arteries and a given stress to your heart. Shoveling the snow off your steps can cause you to experience angina. The pain is predictable in terms of its severity, how long it lasts, and what brings about relief (such as a single tablet of nitroglycerin placed under the tongue). On the other hand, unstable angina describes a new pattern of pain not previously experienced, for example, pain previously felt after a flight of stairs is now suddenly experienced at rest. Unstable angina is a medical emergency that should be immediately evaluated by a doctor.In many instances during an angina attack your EKG, (a tracing of the electrical activity of your heart) may show signs of cardiac injury. However, it is also possible that your EKG can be completely normal, and this finding does not rule out heart attack or angina. If you are having chest pain and your EKG appears normal, your doctor may do an echocardiogram or administer radioactive dye and do a heart perfusion study. Your doctor may take a sample of your blood to have it analyzed for any elevations of your heart enzymes.

If you have heart muscle damage, the injured tissue will release chemicals called isoenzymes. If these heart isoenzymes are increased, this may be a sign that you are having a heart attack. If you have a history of risk factors for coronary artery disease and if your symptoms are stable, your doctor may do a pharmacologic stress test. A dobutamine echocardiogram study may be done. You will be given a drug that will increase your heart rate. You will be monitored with a continuous EKG to see if there are any changes on your EKG that suggest decreased perfusion to your heart muscles. Occasionally your cardiologist may want to do a coronary angiogram, which is a test that uses a dye to assess the extent of your coronary artery disease.

A chest pain syndrome that may be more prevalent in women is an entity called syndrome X. If you have this syndrome, you may have an exaggerated response of the small arteries that go to your heart muscles. This exaggerated response is constriction of the diameter of your arteries. When this happens, you have decreased blood flow going to your heart. Usually women that suffer from this illness have a generalized increase in their body pain overall. This disease is undergoing further research at present. The prevalence of the cardiac syndrome X is higher in women when compared to men. Estrogen deficiency has been shown to play a major role in the origin of cardiac syndrome X. Aspirin can affect your blood's ability to clot and, if you are having angina or if you suspect that you are having a heart attack, aspirin can be lifesaving. Nutrients such as fish oils might be effective for the prevention of heart disease. Remember that angina (heart pain) is not a heart attack. Angina is your body's warning to you that something is wrong and only means that some of your heart muscle is not getting enough blood temporarily.

Angina does not mean that your heart muscle is suffering permanent damage. A heart attack, on the other hand, occurs when the blood flow to your heart muscle is suddenly and permanently cut off. This event will usually cause permanent damage to your heart muscle. If you have angina, you must assume that you have underlying coronary artery disease unless proven otherwise. If you have unstable angina or chest pain at rest, you may need hospitalization for intensive medical therapy. Aspirin and heparin can be given to decrease the clotting factors of your bloodstream. If you have angina, these drugs can decrease the progression of angina to a heart attack.

If you suspect that you are having a heart attack, seek immediate medical attention. Most deaths associated with an acute heart attack occur during the first hours following the onset of the heart attack. Nitroglycerine and morphine might be administered to you through your veins. If your heart rate is abnormal, your cardiologist will treat your abnormal heart rate as well. Your EKG can be sent by telemetry by your emergency medical technician to a local emergency room so that the emergency room doctor can make a diagnosis of your heart rhythm and recommend any treatments that may be immediately necessary. It is important that blood is restored to your heart muscle. Sometimes your blood flow to your heart muscles can be increased by administering therapy to you that will break up blood clots in your heart blood vessels. Streptokinase is one drug that can be used in this situation. You will be confined to bed for 24 to 36 hours. You will be placed in a cardiac care unit. Your activities will be gradually increased. There are enzymes that are released into your bloodstream when you have heart muscle damage.

Other medicines called as beta blockers can be used to slow your heart rate and decrease the contraction of your heart muscles. This maneuver will conserve oxygen. Propanolol (Inderal) is an example of a beta blocker. Calcium channel blockers (Verapimil) affect the calcium in your muscle cells. Calcium channel blockers such as Verapamil can decrease the incidence of you having angina as well as a heart attack. If medication fails to control your angina, coronary artery bypass surgery is sometimes necessary. A blood vessel is grafted onto your blocked artery. This allows your blood flow to bypass the blockage so that blood can go to your heart muscle to provide your heart muscle with needed oxygen. Your surgeon can use an artery inside your chest or take a vein from your leg. Another treatment that can be used to increase your artery size is called balloon angioplasty. This involves insertion of a catheter that has a tiny balloon on the end of it into an artery either in your arm or your leg. The balloon is inflated briefly to widen your vessel in places where your arteries are narrow.

Another type of procedure that can increase your blood flow to your heart is called a stent. A stent is a surgical procedure, but it is a minor procedure compared to open-heart surgery. Stents are implanted through your veins with a catheter. The stent expands when it is placed. The stent will provide better blood flow at the location of your artery where the blood flow is decreased. The purpose of the stent is to permanently hold your artery open. There are three other causes of non-cardiac chest pain that you should be familiar with; intercostal neuropathy, costochondritis and Tsetse's syndrome. Injury to your nerve under your rib bone can occur following a rib fracture, lung surgery or heart surgery or from an infection. This pain may be relieved by anticonvulsant and/or antidepressant drugs. In some instances, your intercostal nerve needs to be injected with a local anesthetic with a steroid. If this fails, freezing the nerve with a cryo probe can provide you with significant pain relief.

Tsetse's syndrome usually occurs in individuals less than 40 years of age. Usually only one pain site is experienced by this syndrome. It occurs at the junction between your ribs and your breastbone (sternum) at the level of your second rib. Costochondritis usually occurs in individuals over 40. More than one area of pain is involved and is at the levels of your second to fifth ribs. Tietze's syndrome follows a respiratory infection while costochondritis follows a neck sprain or coronary heart disease. The treatment of these two pain syndromes is the same as the intercostal neuropathy with the exception that injection therapy is done at the location of the pain. Chest pain must not be ignored. In most cases it is benign. However, in some instances, it is fatal. You must therefore seek medical attention if you experience chest pain.

# 30. ABDOMINAL PAIN

Pain in your abdomen bladder and kidney can be disabling and severe. Abdominal pain in general occurs more often in women than in men. Stress, diet, and the work environment may be causes of abdominal pain in general. Various abdominal pains can occur in your upper, mid, or lower abdomen. Cramping and intermittent pain is easily caused by disorders of your bowel, gallbladder, and ureter of your kidney or your fallopian tubes from your uterus. Pain in your abdomen and pelvis is called visceral pain and is non-specific with respect to the exact location of your pain. Many nerves from many organs can send pain signals to your spinal cord and brain. Your brain can affect the nerves in your stomach and cause you to have an upset stomach. For example, if you are anxious or have to give a speech in front of a large crowd, you may develop "butterflies" in your stomach. You might feel the effect of your stress within your gastrointestinal system. If you are facing a stressful situation, your brain can influence specialized cells in your gastrointestinal system called mast cells to release histamine.

A common syndrome in adults is the irritable bowel syndrome (IBS), which is frequently diagnosed in the general population. Approximately 30 percent of patients seen by gastroenterologists suffer from IBS. It is more common in women and may even be seen in adolescents. If you have IBS, this disease can impair your quality of life. The exact cause of IBS remains to be discovered. IBS can be caused by physiological, psychological, and behavioral factors. Sometimes you may have severe symptoms without any physical findings. This pain is not confined to one area of your gut but it is global over your stomach. Sometimes IBS is diagnosed in patients who suffer from fibromyalgia. Pain associated with IBS can be caused by depression or other behavioral illnesses. If you have psychosocial factors, these factors can influence the frequency of your symptoms as well as the severity of your symptoms. If you suffer from IBS, you may have a previous history of physical, sexual, or emotional abuse. Usually extensive diagnostic tests are not utilized for your doctor to diagnose your IBS because there are no definitive tests for this disease. The criterion for the diagnosis of IBS is difficult because of the variety of physical complaints associated with IBS. If you have moderate symptoms, you may require psychological treatment and occasionally pharmacologic management.

Histamine makes the nerves in your gastrointestinal system contract the smooth muscle in your gut. This will cause you to have cramps. It can also cause you to have diarrhea is some instances. The new drug Lotronex (alosetron) is used to treat abdominal pain and discomfort as well as any symptoms of diarrhea. Lotronex is the first drug approved by the FDA to be used for IBS treatment. Another new drug designed to treat IBS that is now unavailable is called Zelnorm (tegaserod). It is a drug that is in a class of medications called gastrointestinal serotonin agonists. This drug is used for the treatment of constipation, bloating, and abdominal pain. Because of serious side effects this drug was withdrawn from the market in March 2007. If you suffer from IBS, you may want to minimize your fat intake. Many foods inhibit your intestinal gas transit. By decreasing the passage of gas through your gastrointestinal system, bloating and the expansion of your bowel can cause you to have pain. Fructose is another food substance that can worsen your IBS symptoms. Fructose is found in honey, fruit, and in some soft drinks. Fructose can cause you to have bloating, cramps, and diarrhea. Bacteria normally live in your digestive system. The bacteria in your colon may use fructose as their food source. In the process of utilizing fructose, hydrogen gas is liberated in your colon from the breakdown of sugars.

Gastro esophageal reflux disease (GERD) can cause burning pain in your lower thorax or your upper abdomen. It is caused by relaxation of the lower esophageal sphincter that allow stomach acid to go into your esophagus. This condition can be treated with ant acids. Upper abdominal pain can come from a hiatal hernia. You may have vomiting as well as generalized abdominal pain. In this condition, your stomach herniates into your chest cavity. You may require surgery to correct this deformity. Abdominal pain can come from ulcers where the lining of your stomach or duodenum is injured or you may have gastritis where the lining of your stomach is inflamed. Treatment for ulcers and gastritis include antacids, H2 blockers like cimetidine and if no relief occurs with these medications the use of protein pump inhibitors like omeprazole (Zegerid) may be therapeutic.

Your pancreas can also be a source of severe pain. The pain in acute situations can radiate from your mid abdomen to your back. Alcohol or a gallstone can injure your pancreas. A lab test that measures your blood amylase level will be abnormal if you have acute pancreatitis. An ultra sound will help in the diagnosis of pancreatic disease. You will need fluid replacement and analgesic medications such as narcotics if you have an acute attack of pancreatitis. Chronic pancreatitis is an inflammation seen usually in chronic alcoholics. The diagnosis is made with a CAT scan or ultrasound or an endoscopic procedure. An appendix or gallbladder inflammation can also be very painful. Your gallbladder is in the upper right side of your abdomen while your appendix is located in the right lower aspect of your abdomen. If either of these organs becomes diseased, you can develop nausea, vomiting and a fever. Surgery may be necessary to remove one of these diseased organs. Laboratory tests, antibiotics and analgesics are necessary. A CAT scan or a HIDA study can be used to diagnose gallbladder disease. Approximately 20 % of patients continue to experience pain post gallbladder surgery. The reason is usually related to a gallstone in the common bile duct. An appendicitis can be diagnosed with an abdominal ultrasound in most cases.

Your immune system can be a cause of abdominal pain. Inflammatory bowel disease is believed to be a disease of your immune system. IBS can respond to diet. However, the inflammatory bowel disease rarely responds to changes in diet. Inflammatory bowel disease includes ulcerative colitis and Crohn's disease. Ulcerative colitis is a chronic disease and a recurrent disease. It involves inflammation of the lining of the colon. It can also involve your rectum. Crohn's disease can involve any part of your gastrointestinal tract, including your mouth all the way to your anus. The causes of Crohn's disease and ulcerative colitis are unknown. Usually inflammatory bowel disease begins in early adult life. However, there are cases reported in the elderly. Genetic factors can make you prone to inflammatory bowel disease. If you have a disorder of your immune system, you are again prone to develop irritable bowel disease. It is possible that your immune system may attack the lining of your gastrointestinal system. Crohn's disease involves the lower ileum (the lowest part of the small intestine). Your rectum can be involved as well. Approximately one third of Crohn's disease patients have their pathology in their colon, whereas one third of patients have their pathology in their ileum and one third have their pathology in both their ileum and colon. The inflammation of your gastrointestinal system can go from the inside of your bowel to the outside.

The inner lining of your gastrointestinal tract can develop ulcers in some cases of Crohn's disease. An ulcer is a break in the lining of the wall of your stomach or small intestine. This break in your gut lining can fail to heal and can be accompanied by inflammation. A fistula from the inside of your bowel to the outside can develop. A fistula is an abnormal communication between a hollow organ and the exterior. With Crohn's disease, you can have fever, diarrhea, pain, and tenderness in the right lower part of your abdomen. You can also develop an abscess around your anus. The inner aspect of your intestine or colon can decrease in diameter, which is called a stricture. If you have Crohn's disease, you can have an increased incidence of gallstones. With Crohn's disease, your bile salts may not be absorbed properly through your ileum. You can also develop kidney stones. You can have a history of frequent liquid bowel movements.

A barium enema is an enema with opaque contrast liquid that outlines your intestines on x-ray images. This test helps your doctor look for abnormalities in your bowel. To examine your lower bowel, your doctor may also use air with the barium to distend your bowel. Through the colonoscope (a flexible fiberoptic instrument), your physician can obtain biopsies of your colon and ilium. If your gastrointestinal system develops an obstruction somewhere in your system, your food cannot pass through this obstruction. You will be treated with fluids through your veins, and a tube will be placed through your nose to suction out substances that are unable to pass through your bowel. Steroids can be necessary to treat the inflammation caused by Crohn's disease. Be aware that chronic cramping, abdominal pain, and diarrhea are noted in both IBS and Crohn's disease.

Ulcerative colitis is another form of inflammatory bowel disease. Ulcerative colitis involves an inflammation of the inner lining of your colon. You will have bloody diarrhea if you have ulcerative colitis. You will have pain in your abdomen. You can develop anemia and the protein in your bloodstream, albumin, will be decreased. A scope in your colon is the key to the diagnosis of your disease. A hernia can cause abdominal pain as well. A hernia is an abnormal protrusion, or bulging out, of part of an organ such as a portion of your intestine through the tissues that normally contain it. In this condition, a weak spot or opening in a body wall, often due to laxity of the muscles, allows part of the organ to protrude causing a hernia to occur. A hernia may develop in almost any part of the body; but the muscles of the abdominal wall are most commonly affected. One major danger of a hernia is that if bowel is contained within the protruding loop it may hinder or stop the blood flow through the intestine (occlusion). More serious still, if the loop itself becomes twisted outside its containing structure, or compressed at the point where it breaks through that structure (a strangulated hernia), the blood supply to the loop will also cease and the entire hernia will undergo tissue death (necrosis). This requires immediate emergency surgery. An umbilical hernia affects both sexes as well. An intestinal loop protrudes through a weakness in the abdominal wall at the navel. A hiatal hernia also affects both sexes. A loop of the stomach when particularly full protrudes upward through the small opening in the diaphragm through which the esophagus passes, thus leaving the abdominal cavity and entering the chest. An incisional hernia is a hernia that occurs at the site of a surgical incision. This is due to strain on the healing tissues due to excessive muscular effort, lifting, coughing, or extreme pressure. Umbilical hernias can be present from birth, but most happen later due to pressure on openings or weaknesses in the abdominal cavity or wall from heavy lifting etc. Hernias tend to run in families, and can be caused by such things as coughing, straining during a bowel movement, lifting heavy objects, accumulation of fluid in the abdominal cavity, and obesity.

The symptoms of hernias vary, depending on the cause and the structures involved. Most begin as small, hardly noticeable breakthroughs. At first, they may be soft lumps under the skin, a little larger than a marble; there usually is no pain. Gradually, the pressure of the internal contents against the weak wall increases, and the size of the lump increases. Early on, the hernia may be reduced which means that the protruding structures can be pushed back into their normal places. If those structures, however, cannot be returned to their normal locations through manipulation, the hernia is said to be irreducible, or incarcerated. The treatment of an incarcerated abdominal hernia is a serious surgical problem. Operations may be marked by high mortality due to the late diagnosis of incarceration and further postoperative complications. For small, non-strangulated and non-incarcerated hernias, various supports and trusses may offer temporary, symptomatic relief. However, the best treatment is surgical closure or repair of the muscle wall through which the hernia protrudes.

Be aware also that compared with patients with aortoiliac occlusive disease, patients with an abdominal aortic aneurysm have a higher frequency of abdominal wall hernia and inguinal hernia, and are at significant increased risk for development of incision hernia postoperatively. The higher frequency of hernia formation in patients with abdominal aoritic aneurysms suggests the presence of a structural defect within the fascia. Further studies are needed to delineate the molecular changes of the aorta and its relation to the abdominal wall fascia. Patients who have had placement of a mesh graft can have lingering severe pain that may become disabling. Chronic inguinodynia or neuralgia after conventional inguinal herniorrhaphy is rare, and diagnosing the exact cause is difficult. Treatment has ranged from local injection to remedial surgery with variable results. The increasing popularity of prosthetic mesh repairs has not eliminated these pain syndromes from occasionally occurring. It appears that coincident neurectomy affords better results than mesh removal alone. Relief with nerve block did not predict favorable outcomes. Despite the popularity and favorable outcomes of prosthetic mesh repairs, persistent postoperative pain still occurs in a small number of patients. This may become more evident with the rising interest in laparoscopy. Correcting this surgery problem, once presented, can be a formidable task. Remedial inguinal with mesh removal and neurectomy will provide relief in selected patients.

Renal stones and kidney stones on occasion can cause abdominal pain in addition to pain in your flanks. Kidney pain can arise from increased pressure in your kidney capsule or in your ureter. Pain you're your ureter can be referred to your sides (flanks) or to your groin. If your kidney is inflamed as from a stone or infection, a punch over the area of your kidney can cause pain. If you have blood in your urine, you may have a stone. If you are a male and if your scrotum is painful and swollen, you need to see your doctor, as you may have twisting of your spermatic cord or torsion of your spermatic cord. You may need surgery. If your scrotum is infected, it is called an epididymitis. Interstitial cystitis is an inflammatory disease of your bladder that can cause you to have lower abdominal pain.

Interstitial cystitis is a painful pelvic pain from the bladder with a cause that is unknown. An examination using a cystoscope by an urologist may reveal ulcerations in the lining of your bladder. The exact cause may be your immune system. Many treatments have been proposed including surgery on your bladder. Psychological treatment may help as well as installation of various substances into your bladder.

Blood vessels in your abdomen may also be a source of abdominal pain. For example, your aorta, which is a major blood vessel that comes off your heart, runs down through your abdomen and divides into major arteries that supply blood flow to your legs. If you have an aneurysm, which is a defect in the wall of this great vessel, you can have pain in your abdomen. An aneurysm needs to be evaluated by your doctor. An aneurysm is a weakness in the wall of your aorta. If you have abdominal pain and are able to feel or palpate a strong pulse in your abdomen you should consult with your physician. This weak area could rupture, which could be fatal. If you can feel a palpable mass in your abdomen this may be an aneurysm. Ask your doctor if the mass that you feel is abnormal.

Your appendix, if it is inflamed, can cause you to have abdominal pain as well. Your appendix is part of your gastrointestinal system. If you have appendicitis, you will have pain in the right lower part of your abdomen. You will experience nausea and vomiting and may have a fever. It is important for you to see a doctor because an untreated appendicitis can rupture and cause peritonitis. Peritonitis can be fatal.

# 31. ELDERLY PAIN

Between the years 2010 and 2030, the population of the United States over 65 years of age will increase by 73%. One out of every five Americans will be over 65 at that time. Between 1900 and 2000, the total US population increased 3 times but the population of people 65 years or older increased more than 10 times. The growth rate for the population 65 years or older is expected to outpace that for the total population during the next several decades. By 2040, the percentage of elderly patients will increase 20%. Elderly patients in the United States are estimated to be 55 million by 2020 and 80 million by 2040. Pain management in elderly patients can be a challenge. Elderly patients can be taking many different medications. Some of these drugs can adversely interact with some pain medications. Senile patients may forget to take their medications as prescribed. Their kidneys do not function as well as in younger patients. Your kidneys are responsible for eliminating drugs. As a result, drugs like morphine can accumulate within an elderly patient's body which could cause an overdose. Your liver metabolizes (breaks down drugs). Some elderly patients cannot afford some medications and therefore do not take them.

Liver function can also be compromised in elderly patients. This decreased function can affect the breakdown of many drugs. An elderly patient's body mass may be decreased as well. As a result, there is less body volume where a drug can go. A younger patient usually has a greater body mass. A dose of drug will be distributed through various body tissues. If you are emaciated, a dose of drug will remain in your blood stream instead of being distributed throughout your body. As a result, the concentration of drug in your blood stream may be higher than expected. With respect to pain management, older patients handle pain medications differently than younger patients. Your kidneys become smaller with age. As a result, there is decreased blood flow to the kidney and less effective filtration with removal of a drug from the kidney. As one ages, the liver undergoes a decrease in mass and blood flow. Decreased saliva noted in some older patients may interfere with swallowing. Drugs prescribed by mouth may be absorbed differently because of changes in stomach acid levels in older patients. The changes in physiology with aging may alter the side effect profile of many drugs.

One other important consideration is that of elderly persons being able to adequately monitor and adhere to their own scheduled pharmacological administration. Elderly patients may skip medication doses or cut them in half. Because pain is very common among the elderly, all elderly patients should be asked about their pain. Chronic pain can lead to depression, and polypharmacy. The cause of an elderly patient's pain may be difficult to identify and may be multifactorial. Inadequate treatment of pain is common among elderly patients. Thus, psychosocial support and nondrug treatments that reduce pain are particularly important. Patient and caregiver education and active caregiver involvement can help reduce pain and improve quality of life. The prevalence of pain in elderly patients is higher among nursing home residents. In elderly patients, the most common sites of pain are joints, and the most common causes of pain are musculoskeletal disorders. Cancer related pain is not infrequent.

Psychological factors such as depression and anxiety can prolong or amplify pain. The effect of age on pain perception is unknown. Perception may be influenced by many sociologic factors. Chronic pain is characterized by a vague onset. The cause is often a chronic disorder. Sometimes the cause is clear, but the pain lasts longer than the expected time for healing. Neuropathic pain often manifests as spontaneous burning pain with superimposed lancinating pain. Neuropathic pain tends to follow the distribution of a neural pathway. Chronic pain in elderly patients may gradually lead to insomnia, decreased appetite, weight loss and constipation. Patients may become preoccupied with physical symptoms, become inactive, and withdraw socially.

Depression is common in older patients. Inactivity can lead to deconditioning. Many elderly patients take pain for granted and do not mention it unless they are asked. The assessment of patients with impaired cognition may be challenging. Patients with dementia may be able to describe their current symptoms but unable to reliably report their previous symptoms. Depression, secondary gain, personality disorders, and psychological stress should be evaluated in all elderly patients. The patient's physical examination should focus on the musculoskeletal system and include palpation for trigger points, evaluation for joint swelling and inflammation, and evaluation for pain with passive range of motion. Pain is suggested by facial grimacing, frowning, or repetitive eye blinking. In the elderly, pain often has multiple causes, and no single predominant cause can be identified. Poor pain management decreases the patient's quality of life and may contribute to suicide. The elderly are more likely than younger patients to experience adverse effects of analgesics. Drug dosing starting low and going upward slowly. Oral analgesic administration is usually preferred because it is convenient and results in relatively steady blood levels.

Acetaminophen is the analgesic of choice for most elderly people with mild to moderate pain. Despite its relative lack of anti-inflammatory activity, acetaminophen is usually the best drug for initial treatment of osteoarthritis. NSAIDs are indicated when inflammation contributes significantly to pain. Adverse effects vary, and a patient may tolerate one NSAID better than another. NSAIDs tend to have a ceiling analgesic dose. The most common adverse effect of all NSAIDs is gastrointestinal upset, which may require stopping the drug. Ulceration and GI bleeding can occur. Ulceration with or without bleeding can occur simultaneously or independently of each other. Risk of ulcers and GI bleeding for people 65 years or over is 3 to 4 times higher than that for middle-aged people. NSAIDs can impair renal function and cause sodium and water retention; they should be used cautiously in the elderly, particularly in those who have a renal disorder. Nonacetylated salicylates may have less renal toxicity and fewer antiplatelet effects than other NSAIDs.

Opioids are the most potent analgesics. Opioids act by blocking receptors in the brain and spinal cord. In the elderly, opioids have an increased half-life and possibly a greater analgesic effect than in younger patients. Nonetheless, the most common error in prescribing these drugs is to give them too infrequently, allowing breakthrough pain. A few opioids have specific advantages and disadvantages in elderly patients. Fentanyl causes less histamine release and thus less vasodilation and hypotension. Meperidine should be avoided in elderly patients. Meperidine is less effective when given orally and can cause confusion; also, it is metabolized to an active form that tends to accumulate and thus may lead to central nervous system excitement and seizures.

Opioid agonist-antagonists, which have both agonist and antagonist effects on opiate receptors, often have psychotomimetic effects in the elderly. As a result, Stadol should not be used in the elderly. In patients with renal insufficiency, excretion of morphine and codeine may be delayed, resulting in undesirably long therapeutic or adverse effects, particularly with sustained-release formulations. In these patients, hydromorphone or oxycodone is less likely to accumulate and may be preferred. Opioids can be given transdermally. However, transdermal fentanyl should be used only in patients who have already been stabilized on opioids. Transdermal fentanyl is long-lasting. The peak analgesic effect of transdermal fentanyl occurs 18 to 24 h after application. If this drug is used, a rapid-onset analgesic is required in the meantime. It is important to know that the reservoir for this system is the skin and not in the patch. If an overdose occurs, removing the patch does little to stop drug delivery within the first 18 h after removal.

Patients must be closely observed if they have a fever. A fever can cause an increased uptake of the drug into the elderly patient's body. As a result an overdose could occur. A heating pad can also cause a fentanyl overdose. Continuous opioid infusion provides steady-state analgesic drug levels. This means that there are no peaks and valleys in the elderly patient's bloodstream. Continuous infusion in palliative care patients may also be useful if regional techniques and NSAIDs are ineffective or inappropriate in patients near the end of life. Patient-controlled analgesia enables a patient to increase drug delivery as needed. This technique results in a more stable blood drug level, thus avoiding the roller-coaster effects of intramuscular dosing. Patient-controlled analgesia reduces overall drug use and has fewer adverse side effects. However, patients with confusion or dementia cannot effectively use patient-controlled analgesia. Opioid muscle injection is rarely used. Initially, drug blood levels are high, resulting in more frequent adverse effects. The blood drug levels decrease rapidly, resulting in pain recurrence.

Unlike NSAIDS, opioids have no ceiling analgesic effect as dosage is increased. The maximum dose is whatever is needed to relieve pain. However, adverse effects may limit the maximum dose that is used. Opioids cause dose-related sedation and respiratory depression. Most elderly patients taking opioids should not drive and should take precautions to prevent falls. Opioids may cause confusion. If confusion is due to an opioid, pupils are usually very constricted. Sometimes decreasing the dose may relieve confusion without significantly decreasing analgesia. If this approach is ineffective, a different analgesic may be necessary. Opioids almost always cause constipation or urinary retention. Patients do not develop tolerance to these adverse effects. When an opioid is started, the patient's intake of fluid and fiber should be increased to try to prevent constipation. If a laxative is needed, a fiber laxative may be used. Movantik may be used for opioid induced constipation. Gabapentin (Neurontin) is frequently prescribed in elderly patients. Dose reductions of gabapentin are recommended in patients with renal insufficiency. Dizziness and drowsiness are common adverse effects. Pregabilin (Lyrica) is frequently in elderly patients with post herpetic neuralgia.

Antidepressant medications are also prescribed as adjunct medications for elderly patients who suffer from pain. The analgesic mechanism of antidepressants involves interruption of brain mechanisms mediated by norepinephrine and serotonin. For tricyclic antidepressants, there is little evidence that one is better than another; however, amitriptyline, which is highly sedating and anticholinergic, should be avoided in the elderly. Calcitonin is a drug that may reduce chronic pain due to osteoporosis. Bisphosphonates can reduce pain due to bone metastasis. Local anesthetics injected into painful muscle areas are sometimes effective. Local anesthetics injected into joints can relieve joint pain. Topical drugs are frequently used for pain originating in peripheral nerves. Capsaicin cream, NSAID creams, or a Lidoderm (lidocaine 5%) patch should be considered as well.

Physical therapy can reduce pain due to musculoskeletal disorders in elderly patients. Aquatic therapy can help muscle and joint pain. Pain due to muscle spasm may be reduced by stretching, muscle massages, cold therapy or heat therapy. Ultrasound therapy may relieve musculoskeletal pain originating in your deep tissues. Transcutaneous electrical nerve stimulation (TENS) can relieve many types of pain as well. Alternative therapies are also used by many patients to control their pain. Occupational therapy can be helpful as well as this modality can teach patients energy saving techniques to be used around their residences.

# 32. GENDER PAIN

The causes and treatments of pain are different for men and women. The study of the differences between how men and women feel pain and are treated for it is a relatively new branch of medicine. Your age, physical design, hormones, psychological issues, and social issues all play a part in why you feel pain. Simply stated, your sex (male or female) is determined by your chromosomes (XX for women, XY for men) and your body's particular anatomy. Your gender (man or woman) is determined by your body's anatomical features and social issues. Gender is an important influence on experiences of clinical and laboratory pain. Women and men differ in their perceptions and experiences of pain. Women as a result of pain neuron electrical, hormonal differences to men are more likely than men to experience recurrent pain, as well as frequent, severe, and longer-lasting pain. Women also tended to experience more pain-related disability and to receive unwarranted psychogenic attributions for pain by health professionals from whom they sought treatment. There are differences in emotional processing of noxious information in men and women and may underlie the gender bias that exists in many chronic pain conditions

Concerning social issues, in most cases men have been programmed since they were children to be macho when dealing with pain. When playing athletic events, boys are often told to "tough it out" when they are hurt. On the other hand, women since childhood have been allowed to express their pain freely. It is socially acceptable for a girl to cry, but it is not so for a boy. Differences between men and women exist with physical characteristics, hormones, and social expectations, just to name a few. One of the reasons men and women feel pain differently has to do with hormones. Sex differences affect the absorption, metabolism (breakdown of drugs), and excretion (elimination of drugs) of many medications. Women respond more favorably to a class of antidepressant medications called serotonin-specific reuptake inhibitors, or SSRIs (for instance, Prozac), than to other antidepressants known as tricyclics (for instance, Elavil).

Sexual differences between men and women are important with respect to drug action, especially because the menstrual cycle can affect the amount of medication in the blood (blood levels). If a female retains fluid, the excess fluid will dilute the action of the drug. Oral contraceptives (for instance, "the pill") can decrease the blood levels of some anticonvulsant medications such as Dilantin. On the other hand, oral contraceptives can increase the blood level of some medications such as Valium. Hormone replacement in women does enhance the effects of antidepressant medications. Approximately two thirds of antidepressant medications in the United States are used by women. Women have more side effects with antidepressant-type medications than men. They suffer more fatigue, gastrointestinal affects, and other adverse effects than men. Gonadal hormonal changes in women that occur monthly (before, during and after the menstrual cycle) alter the metabolism (breakdown of drugs in the liver) of certain drugs and can affect their removal from the body. One of the reasons why men and women differ in the perception of pain results from the effects of the female hormones estrogen and progesterone on the brain and spinal cord (the nervous system). The effects of the menstrual cycle on the nervous system vary before, during, and after menses. In the future, sexual and/or gender differences may allow a doctor to individualize treatments that are specific for each sex. It has also been found that low testosterone in males can also lower the pain threshold. The wiring of the central nervous system is influenced by differences in sex.

Male and female brains have approximately the same number of receptors for estrogen and androgen. Estrogen is primarily a female hormone, whereas androgen is primarily a male hormone. A receptor is an area on the outer covering, or membrane, of a cell where hormones or drugs attach and start to take action. The way receptors respond to drugs and hormones effects the body's response to both drugs and hormones. For example, giving estrogen to a man does not affect his brain like it does a woman. In the same way, giving androgens (male hormones) to a female brain does not cause the same response as in a male. Researchers have therefore concluded that hormone and hormonal receptor differences between men and women also influence the regulation and transmission of the nervous impulses that transmit pain. Estrogen (the female hormone) affects the central nervous system levels of dopamine and serotonin, which are involved with mood disorders. Women experience more depression than males. Men may have more serotonin receptors, which may be a reason why they suffer from a lower incidence of depression. As a result, a woman's greater sensitivity to pain may be dependent on the fact that she has less serotonin in the brain and spinal cord.

Pain perception will vary from person to person. While, men and women report the same number of negative (or adverse) reactions during and following treatment with therapeutic medications, negative effects of medicines are higher and more serious in women than in men. This disparity may be influenced by the fact that women use medications more often than men and in different doses, and because the different ways the drugs are absorbed, metabolized (broken down), and removed from the body by men and women. Women often report more migraine headaches and arthritic pain than men. Women also have a greater discomfort for the same type of pain than men and are more likely to develop long-term pain after an injury. Women also use more over-the-counter pain medications and have more doctor visits than men. Media advertising often recommends a certain medication for a specific condition, but none of the advertisements discuss doses with respect to the body size of a man or woman. Body size determines the amount of a medicine needed to treat a painful condition. Take a look at an aspirin bottle label. Does it tell you the dosage for a man or woman?

In 1977, the U.S. Food and Drug Administration (FDA) prohibited women of child-bearing age from being involved in clinical trials. As a result, many drug studies were done only on men until recently. In 1985, a U.S. public health service task force addressed the Department of Health and Human Services and expressed the need to establish a policy that included women in clinical drug studies. In 1990, the Government Accounting Office issued a report and concluded that there was a lack of compliance in including women in clinical drug trials. In 1993, Congress made it mandatory that women, as well as minorities, be included in clinical drug trials. Also in 1993, the FDA began allowing women of child-bearing age to take part in clinical drug trials. In 1994, the National Institutes of Health issued guidelines to grant applications to confirm that researchers complied with the inclusion of women of child-bearing age in their studies.

The anatomic differences between men and women also influence their reactions to medications. In general, women have lower body weights and organ sizes and a higher percentage of body fat, factors that need to be taken into account when discussing the way the body handles drugs and their use in men and women. For example, the muscle relaxant Valium (diazepam) causes more impairment of voluntary muscle control in women than in men, probably because of lower body weight of women as compared to men. Differences in drug reactions are caused by differences in the way men and women process drugs. The transport of drugs within the blood-stream and the chemicals that break down drugs differ in men and women. Enzymes in the liver assist breaking down drugs. One of these enzymes is the CYP 3A4 liver enzyme. This enzyme breaks down more than 50 percent of all therapeutic drugs. In women, drugs that have been metabolized in the liver are delivered more slowly to the bloodstream, where they are then sent to the kidneys for excretion from the body.

Because more of the pain medications are not taken out of the liver, a higher concentration of these drugs in the liver requires processing. The liver enzymes in women have to process higher concentrations of the drugs than males. Liver enzymes in women may also not metabolize the antidepressants of the selective serotonin-specific reuptake inhibitor class. Women have a lower stomach acid secretion than men. This can increase the absorption of drugs such as Elavil or Valium, and decrease the absorption of acidic drugs such as Dilantin and barbiturates. Women weigh less than men and have a lower total blood value than men. Body fat is 11 percent higher in women between the ages of 25 and 35. After a drug is absorbed from either the stomach or the small intestine, the drug is distributed throughout the tissues in the body.

Drugs that have a high affinity for fat are called fat-soluble drugs. If an individual has a high body fat content, some drugs may rapidly enter the fatty tissue. This action will decrease the level of medication in the blood and make it less effective. However, if repetitive administration of a drug causes a high concentration of that drug in body fat, it will eventually be released back into the bloodstream, which can cause a significantly higher blood level of the drug at that time. The liver breaks down and eliminates most drugs. Biologic systems, including the liver, may be more efficient in men than in women. Drugs may be eliminated from the body more effectively by the kidneys in men when compared to women. As a result, equal doses of medication could result in a higher blood level of that particular drug in a woman than in a man. This in turn could cause serious side- effects in the woman but not in the man. Men and women differ with respect to their response to medications. Note, therefore, that the dosage for men and women must differ. However, many doctors are unaware of the gender-specific differences between men and women with respect to their responses to medications, as well as the differences between men and women with respect to body weight. An obese woman may require more medication to achieve the same pain relief than a thin woman.

The way in which antidepressant medications are absorbed, distributed in the bloodstream, and eliminated by the kidneys differs in men and women. Monthly hormone cycles in women can influence the effects of some antidepressants. Further, oral contraceptives and hormones can alter drug interactions in women. For example, acetaminophen (Tylenol) is made inactive in women taking oral contraceptives when compared to women who are not taking oral contraceptives. High blood levels of estradiol (a female hormone) sensitize a female to thermal (heat) pain. Premenopausal women take longer to empty stomach content such as food and medication. In essence, this means that medications in the stomach are slower to leave the stomach to go into the small intestine. The small intestine has a greater absorptive capacity than the stomach. If a medication is delayed in passage from the stomach to the small intestine, medicine will be absorbed more slowly into the blood. Consequently, the blood level of the drug may be decreased.

A question that has yet to be answered is why many medications come in one single dose. This chapter relates that men and women differ in their responses to drugs. One would therefore expect that some drugs would be packaged in doses for men and doses for women. Furthermore, there should be differences in drug doses for thin and obese patients.

# Index

abdominal aortic aneurysm 177

Action potentials 4

Addiction 38, 41, 43, 44

A-delta fibers 4

alodynia 147

androgen 188

Animal models 15

ankylosing spondylitis 47, 132, 133

Anticonvulsant drugs 7, 57, 59

anti-depressant drugs 63

antispasticity medications 54

appendicitis 27, 156, 175, 179

Beriberi 126

Biofeedback 23, 91, 98

Burger's 154

C fibers 4, 6, 46, 71

Calcitonin 139, 185

causalgia 147

chicken pox 141

Clonidine 76, 150

clonidine patch 76, 151

computer 9, 1, 2, 3, 6, 7, 9, 10, 11, 15, 18, 19, 21, 27, 28, 31, 35, 51, 63, 82, 124

diary 80

disc herniations 95

dorsal column stimulator 23, 145, 151

drug seekers 42, 43

Electromyography 28, 29

EMG 28, 29, 113

EMLA 72, 73

enkephalins 6, 22, 23

Erythemalgia 155

Estrogen 134, 169, 188

facet joint 82

fat-soluble drugs 190

fentanyl 38, 70, 74, 75, 76, 164, 183, 184

GERD 174

Gout 133, 134

headaches 31, 39, 42, 48, 54, 59, 61, 66, 72, 85, 92, 102, 110, 115, 116, 117, 118, 119, 120, 121, 155, 189

Hypnosis 23, 92

inguinodynia 178

internuncial fibers 5

Interstitial cystitis 178

irritable bowel syndrome 103, 173

Ketamine 74

Kyphyplasty 139

Lidoderm patch 76, 144

Liver enzymes 190

Menthol 72

mexiletine 125

migraine headache 60, 117, 118

myofascial pain 109, 110, 111, 112, 113

narcotic 156

Narcotic drugs 7, 35

neuroma 150

NSAIDs 45, 46, 48, 49, 74, 183, 184

nucleus pulposus, 96, 97, 100

osteoarthritis 46, 47, 48, 71, 99, 129, 130, 131, 132, 183

osteoporosis 26, 45, 79, 137, 138, 139, 185

Pain perception 188

Pain signals 4

Pinzmetal's angina 168

Polyarteritis nodosa 157

post-herpetic neuralgia 66, 141, 142, 143, 144

post-herpetic neuralgia are 20 percent 142

prostatism 163

Raynaud's 153

Raynaud's phenomenon 153

Raynaud's 153

rheumatoid arthritis 25, 46, 47, 48, 55, 71,
    72, 79, 99, 104, 105, 115, 129, 131,
    132, 133, 154, 157

scleroderma 153, 154, 156

syndrome X 169

Systemic lupus erythematosus 157

Temporal arteritis 155

Tietze's syndrome 171

topical analgesics 69, 72

topical capsaicin 71

Transmission 5

trigger points 109, 110, 111, 112, 113, 182

ultrasound 81

Uric acid 133, 134

Vascular 153

Vertebroplasty 139

Whiplash 101

Zanaflex 52, 54, 55

# About the Author

Dr. Ackerman is a clinician, academician, lecturer, author, researcher, and an expert witness in pain management medical malpractice cases. Dr. Ackerman is: Board Certified in both Pain Medicine and Anesthesiology, is a Graduate of the University Of Louisville School Of Medicine. He did a residency in anesthesiology at the University of Kentucky, and was Chief Resident in Anesthesiology and Critical Care Medicine and he did a Fellowship in Pain Medicine at the Texas Tech Health Sciences Center in Lubbock, Texas. Dr. Ackerman was: Nominated previously for the Southern Medical Society Medical Research Award, Bristol-Meyers Squibb award for distinguished achievement in Pain Research was a recipient of the Karl Koehler research grant from the American Society of Regional Anesthesia and Pain Medicine.

He has been a guest speaker at medical school department meetings workman's Compensation meetings and academic symposiums throughout the country and at international meetings. His research has been featured in the National media. He published sixteen books and many chapters in multiple medical textbooks including the AMA best seller: The AMA Guides to Injury and Disease Causation (First and Second editions). He authored 136 scientific articles in prestigious medical journals such as: Anesthesia Analgesia, Canadian Journal of Anaesthesia, Regional Anesthesia and Pain Management, The Journal of Hand Surgery etc.

He was a Lt. Col in the US Army and Chief of Anesthesiology of two Army Medical Center Hospitals and was director of pain management at two private hospitals. He was an Emergency Room physician at the Ireland Army Hospital at Fort Knox, Kentucky. Dr. Ackerman was Director of Pain Management at a University Hospital pain clinic and was an Associate Professor as well as an attending clinical instructor in critical care and hyperbaric medicine as well as Director of Obstetric Anesthesia at the University of Kentucky. He was director of pain management at two private hospitals and was selected to "Who's Who in International Medicine". He is now in private practice and is president of his medical clinic. He has a strong belief in medical ethics and the prevention of medical fraud.

www.ingramcontent.com/pod-product-compliance
Lightning Source LLC
Chambersburg PA
CBHW050209230526
45470CB00001B/306